Minimal Brain Dysfunction: Fact or Fiction

Advances in Biological Psychiatry

Vol. 1

S. Karger · Basel · München · Paris · London · New York · Sydney

Symposium on Minimal Brain Dysfunction, Amsterdam, April 1977

Minimal Brain Dysfunction: Fact or Fiction

Editors
A.F. Kalverboer; H.M. van Praag, Groningen, and
J. Mendlewicz, Bruxelles

2 figures and 5 tables, 1978

S. Karger · Basel · München · Paris · London · New York · Sydney

Advances in Biological Psychiatry

In preparation
Vol. 2: Childhood Psychopharmacology: Current Concepts.
J. Mendlewicz (Bruxelles) ed., and *H.M. van Praag* (Groningen) ed.
ISBN 3–8055–2901–5

Cataloging in Publication
Minimal brain dysfunction: fact or fiction
Editors: A.F. Kalverboer, H.M. van Praag, and J. Mendlewicz. – Basel, New York, Karger, 1978.
(Advances in biological psychiatry, v.1)
1. Minimal Brain Dysfunction I. Kalverboer, Alex, Fedde, ed. II. Praag, Herman Meir van, ed. III. Mendlewicz, J., ed. IV. Title V. Series
W1 AD44 v.1/WL 340.3 M665
ISBN 3–8055–2864–7

Printed in Switzerland by Thür AG Offsetdruck, Pratteln
ISBN 3–8055–2864–7

Contents

Adv. biol. Psychiat., vol. 1, p. 1 (Karger, Basel 1978)

Opening Remarks

First of all, I would like to welcome all the participants to this symposium and extend my gratitude to the organisers and sponsors of this conference.

I particularly would like to take this opportunity to acknowledge the contribution of Dr. *Bruinvels* who has helped us without limits in his capacity of secretary of the Society for many years.

In the name of the Society, I also wish to thank the invited lecturers and discussants who gave us the benefit of their experience.

It is a privilege and an honor to be able to serve the Society of Biological Psychiatry after Prof. *Van Praag*'s chairmanship for more than a decade. *Van Praag* is an example for all of us who are interested in the field of Biological Psychiatry, not only because of the quality and originality of his work (with which most of us happen to be familiar, but much more, as I see it, because of the spirit and drive he is giving to promote the development of this discipline.

In the name of all of us, I want to thank Prof. *Van Praag* for the devotion he has shown and is still showing to our Society. This may sound like postmortem eulogies, but, fortunately for all of us, *Van Praag* is still a young man and I am certain we will continue to benefit from his major contributions.

Our symposium is devoted to what has been called the Minimal Brain Dysfunction (MBD) syndrome and, as in many behavioral topics, there are facts and fiction, which I hope we will be able to discuss without expecting to elucidate the various problems raised by the MBD syndrome in terms of nosology, etiology and treatment. Although there have been many conferences and publications lately on this subject, we are still lacking a unified conceptual model and treatment programme for the MDB syndrome. Our meeting should bring us the latest viewpoints on MBD from various disciplines such as psychology, neurology, psychiatry, pharmacology and epidemiology, represented by top experts in these fields.

I look forward to the sessions with great interest and with the desire to learn something from this conference.

J. Mendlewicz, MD, PhD, Chairman

Adv. biol. Psychiat., vol. 1, pp. 2–4 (Karger, Basel 1978)

Introduction

H.M. van Praag

Department of Biological Psychiatry, Psychiatric University Clinic, Groningen

Is minimal brain dysfunction (MBD) fact or fiction? Of course it is a fact. Who would want to refute that the functional integrity of the brain can be slightly disturbed. Is MBD as a diagnostic entity fact or fiction? This is a controversial question, which is not surprising because MBD is an ill-defined notion, vague and, therefore, multi-interpretable. Let me discuss a few causes of this vagueness.

First of all, the term MBD is used in two different meanings: symptomatological and aetiological. In the former case the term practically denotes the hyperkinetic syndrome. The term is then regarded as applicable to children who are hyperactive and easily distracted, whose performance at school is below par and whose frustration tolerance is low. In this usage, the term MBD indicates a syndrome, regardless of the question whether irregularities in brain function are or are not demonstrable.

Others consider the diagnosis MBD when behaviour disorders – be they hyperkinetic or of a different nature – are observed in combination with slight neurological and/or EEG disorders, which are accepted as incontrovertible evidence of some disturbance of brain function. The exact nature of the neurological and/or EEG disorders considered characteristic of this diagnosis, is not specified; and this has opened the door to diagnostic chaos.

Otherwise, it is not exceptional in psychiatry that a particular term is used in an aetiological meaning in some cases, but symptomatologically in others. This, of course, is just asking for confusion. A typical example in this context is the neurosis concept. By this I only mean to say that mishandling of a concept, as for example the MBD concept, is by no means an exception.

The *second* source of confusion is closely related to the first. What is the origin of the behaviour disorders commonly associated with the MBD concept? Minimal brain dysfunction of course, one might be inclined to say. However, the hyperkinetic syndrome is sometimes observed in individuals who show not the slightest sign of disturbed brain function and, on the other hand, evidence of (slightly) disturbed brain function can be found in individuals without any hyperkinetic symptom. Hyperkinetic symptoms are more or less physiological in young children who are tired. On the other hand, they can be the resultant of neurotically disturbed family relations; they can be observed in psychotic children, and can also be associated with severe morphological brain lesions. Finally, there are indications that genetic factors, too, can contribute to the development of the hyperkinetic syndrome.

In brief; the behaviour disorders commonly associated with MBD are far from specific. On the contrary. They constitute an aetiologically non-specific syndrome. They *may* be related to MBD, but they can equally well be due to causative factors of a quite different nature (Fish, 1971).

The *last* factor which has caused confusion is the pharmacotherapy of hyperkinetic children. Amphetamine derivatives have come to occupy a prominent position in this therapy, especially in the USA. They are believed to reduce distractibility and hyperactivity and to lead to better organized behaviour and better performance at school. This effect has been described as paradoxical for, after all, one would rather have expected an anti-therapeutic, disorganizing effect of central stimulants.

Is this paradoxical effect fact or fiction? In some cases it is a well-documented fact (*van Praag,* 1977). In other cases these agents are ineffective. We do not know why. Psychological factors might play a role. It is conceivable, for example, that neurotic hyperkinesia responds less well to amphetamines than organic hyperkinesia. Or are the differences biochemically determined? Can disorganization of different biochemical systems lead to the same (hyperkinetic) syndrome? If so, then it would be thinkable that a given type of agent has a therapeutic effect in one case, but not in the other.

So much for a few of the factors which have made the twin concepts MBD and hyperkinetic syndrome so confusing, and which have persuaded us to devote a symposium to them. There were positive arguments as well, for the MBD concept raises fascinating questions. One such question is: what is the basis of the therapeutic effect of amphetamines? Amphetamines enhance central catecholaminergic activity. If anything, potentiation of motor hyperactivity could have been expected on this basis (*van Praag,* 1978). The hypothesis has been advanced that the central nervous system in children with hyperkinetic symptoms is underaroused, and that their behaviour might be compared with that of children who are overtired. An interesting hypothesis, but efforts to test it have so far hardly been made.

Another question which arises in this context concerns the fate of hyperkinetic children who outgrow childhood. Amphetamine medication is rarely continued beyond adolescence. Do the symptoms disappear, or can this syndrome be observed in adults also? Or is it replaced by other behaviour disorders?

Again, we do not know. Very few follow-up studies have so far been made (*Weiss et al.*, 1971; *Menkes et al.*, 1967; *Mendelson et al.*, 1971). Some investigators found pathological features at a later age in a large percentage of cases; others were unable to confirm this. However, the groups studied were small, and in so heterogeneous a category this can easily lead to erroneous conclusions.

General discontent about this confusion combined with an interest in the mishandled concepts provided the arguments for broaching the subject of the twin concepts of MBD and hyperkinetic syndrome today. This symposium is the 20th in the series, and to me it is one of special significance because, today, I resigned my membership of the board of the Society. I cannot deny that I take this step with a heavy heart. I was one of the founders of the Society in 1966, and have been its president these 11 years – a long period during which the successive boards have tried to arouse interest in and understanding for the field of activity and the problem definitions of biological psychiatry.

I resign with some sadness, but also with confidence. With confidence because the new president will be *Julien Mendlewicz:* a good psychiatrist, a good researcher and a good organizer. I can do nothing else, and nothing better, than wish him and his fellow members of the board every success, from the bottom of my heart.

References

Borland, B.L. and Heckmann, H.K.: Hyperactive boys and their brothers. Archs gen. Psychiat. *33:* 669–675 (1976).

Cantwell, D.P.: Psychiatric illness in the families of hyperactive children. Archs gen. Psychiat. *27:* 414–417 (1972).

Fish, B.: The 'one child, one drug' myth of stimulants in hyperkinesis. Archs gen. Psychiat. *25:* 193–198 (1971).

Mendelson, W.; Johnson, N., and Stewart, M.: Hyperactive children as teenagers. A follow-up study. J. nerv. ment. Dis. *153:* 272–279 (1971).

Menkes, M.; Rowe, J., and Menkes, J.: A 25-year follow-up study on the hyperkinetic child with minimal brain dysfunction. Pediatrics, Springfield *39:* 393–399 (1967).

Praag, H.M. van: The significance of dopamine for the pathogenesis of schizophrenia and the mode of action of antipsychotic drugs. Br. J. Psychiat. *130:* 463–474 (1977).

Praag, H.M. van: Psychotropic drugs. A guideline for the practitioner (Bruner/Mazel, New York, in press, 1978).

Weiss, G.; Minde, K.; Werry, J.S.; Douglas, V., and Nemeth, E.: Studies on the hyperactive child. Five year follow-up. Archs gen. Psychiat. *24:* 409–414 (1971).

Dr. *H.M. van Praag*, Psychiatric University Clinic, Department of Biological Psychiatry, Oostersingel 59, *Groningen* (The Netherlands)
Present address: Psychiatric University Clinic, Utrecht (The Netherlands)

Adv. biol. Psychiat., vol. 1, pp. 5–17 (Karger, Basel 1978)

MBD: Discussion of the Concept

Alex F. Kalverboer

Laboratory for Experimental Clinical Psychology, Department of Clinical Psychology, State University, Groningen

Introduction

One of the most remarkable clinical concepts is that of MBD, originally indicating 'minimal brain damage', at present 'minimal brain dysfunction', and possibly in the near future 'maximal brain damage', at least if we follow *Towbin* (1971), who states 'all of us have a touch of cerebral palsy'. The term MBD is generally used to identify school-aged children within the normal range of intelligence, who present behaviour and/or learning problems which are assumed to be connected with 'minimal' CNS dysfunction. Terms such as over- or hyperactivity, short attention span, and lack of concentration, impulsivity, lability of mood, and irritability purport to describe disorders in the behavioural organization, frequently observed in such children, while deficits in the perception and integration of spatial and temporal relationships are also often reported usually in connection with reading and/or writing difficulties. 'Soft' neurological signs, such as minor deficiencies in motor co-ordination, reflex asymmetries, mild visual or hearing impairments, dyskinesia's (such as choreiform jerks, athetoid movements), general clumsiness, poor fine or gross visuo-motor co-ordination, and signs of a delayed motor development are also frequently part of the syndrome. Few problem areas have evoked as much interest in specialists of such widely varying disciplines as physics, psychology, education and biochemistry, as the MBD 'syndrome'. At the same time, however, hardly any concept in the clinical nomenclature has occasioned so much controversy and confusion. What has led to this broad interest and what is the background of the confusion and controversy?

History of the Concept

In order to better understand the present situation it may be helpful to briefly retrace the history of the concept. The wide interest in the MBD problem is partly due to convergences in educational, psychological and medical thinking during the last 50 years, attended by refinements of methods and techniques for assessment and guidance in each of these disciplines.

In the field of education there was a shift from subject-centered to child-centered teaching. Commencing in the early years of this century new guiding principles for the teacher developed from painstaking observations of the child's free exploration of his physical environment (Montessory, Decroly) and from reflexion on his social activity (Parkhurst). The child came to be considered as an active individual, who learned by exploration (Montessori) and who should be confronted with 'meaningful structures' (Decroly). Gestalt psychology in particular profoundly influenced educational practices.

Educational thinking was influenced not only by general 'laws' concerning the child's mental development, but also by a concern for individual abilities and limitations, leading to the foundation of special schools for children with learning problems. Initially, criteria for the selection of children requiring special consideration were crude, but they gradually became more refined and objective, not least as a result of important developments in the field of psycho-diagnostics. Starting with Binet in 1905 who was required to find a method that would discriminate between lazy and incapable children, psycho-metric methods became increasingly helpful in the determination of the most suitable learning environment for the child. Originally, intelligence tests were assumed to indicate the child's 'general intellectual potential'. Only gradually more relativistic opinions on the value of test scores developed. Children were crudely categorized as mentally deficient or mentally defective, backwards, subnormal or slow learning, normal, gifted or superior, labels which were adapted to the available resources.

Reflecting the growing complexity of the society, schools made increasing demands on their pupils: knowledge of the traditional skills and tools was no longer sufficient for the child; he should be able to find intelligent solutions for new problems. These more complex scholastic standards, the refinement in diagnostic tools and the development of institutions for special education led to the identification of groups of children with learning problems, previously unrecognized or not manifesting themselves.

After approximately 1940, interest in specific learning and behavioural disorders that might relate to basic deficits in perceptual, perceptuo-motor or cognitive functions considerably increased. At the theoretical level, by far the most important contribution was made by Piaget, who developed a differentiated theory on the integration of 'organic' (motor, sensory-motor) and mental (spatial-constructive, cognitive) functions during human ontogeny. There was a growing knowledge and recognition of the essential role of the child's 'organismic make up' in the development of his adaptation to the social and physical environment. Specific learning problems were attributed to basic defects in the integration of motor and perceptual information.

At about the same time of these developments in education and psychology there was a considerable change in neuropsychological thinking, which evolved from the previous 'mechanistic' and 'connectionistic' models to the idea that the nervous system functions as a differentiated whole in continuous interaction with the environment (*Boring,* 1960). *Lashley* is one of the first representatives of this theoretical movement, which owes much to Gestalt psychology (*Beach et al.*, 1960). The nervous system is considered as 'a composite of many interacting systems' and *Lashley* expresses the view that 'the nets active in rhythmic and spatial organization are apparently almost co-extensive with the nervous system' (*Lashley,* 1930, 1951). Although a certain functional differentiation is not denied, it is the essence of the theory that the organism acts as a whole: 'within certain regions of the brain with relatively specific functions (e.g. the visual cortex) there exists equipotentiality' (*Lashley,* 1950). *Lashley* and followers consider temporal and spatial integration of perception and motor activity as the essential function of the CNS (*Lashley,* 1958). Contemporary neuropsychological thinking as exemplified by *Luria* (1973) considers the CNS as a totally active, integrated system, responsible for the refined adaptation of the behaviour to environmental variations. Diffuse damage to the cerebrum may particularly lead to disorders in the organization of complex behaviour, such as those described in so-called MBD children.

There is a remarkable similarity in Piaget's and Lashley's thinking, indicated by their common view that in all activities the organism is totally involved. *Lashley* gives the example of the perception of verticality, whereby information about changes in position and motion in the visual field must be continuously integrated with information about the body posture and the tonic activity in the muscles.

Developments in clinical thinking underly some current views on neurobehavioural relationships in children. Briefly traced, these developments are the following:

Firstly, there is the effect that descriptions of phenomena associated with demonstrable brain pathology in adults have had on thinking about developmental disturbances. The 'aphasia' literature in particular, focussing attention on disorders in receptive and expressive language in relation to brain disorder has affected the development of the MBD concept.

Disorders in the acquisition of spoken and written language become considered as analogues of such aphasic phenomena in adults (*Strother,* 1973). When hard evidence for brain damage is lacking in children presenting such developmental disorders, the label MBD is generally used to suggest the organic background. Although earlier terms, such as developmental 'aphasia' and developmental 'agraphia' were gradually replaced by more neutral ones, such as 'dyslexia' and 'linguistic retardation', such dysfunctions still remained to be considered as signs of CNS disorder, even when independent neurological evidence was lacking (*Strother,* 1973; *Wedell,* 1973). A similar development occurred in connection with other phenomena related to adult brain pathology, such as 'functional retrogression' and 'loss of abstract reasoning ability'. By analogy developmental delays and persistent concrete modes of thinking became also in themselves considered as signs of CNS disorder, although it was realized that developmental disorders were different from signs of functional disintegration in brain-damaged adults.

There is a significant number of children, who have severe difficulties in acquiring spoken and written language, unaccountable for on the basis of lack of intelligence, primary sensory, motor and emotional disorders, or lack of environmental stimulation. MBD becomes a usual 'diagnosis' for such cases, as well as for children presenting unexplained discrepancies between the 'actual' level of performance and the assumed potential.

Another important influence on the development of the MBD concept has been descriptions of the behavioural consequences of known brain damage in children. As typical symptoms in children after encephalitis (*Hohman,* 1922; *Bond,* 1932) and after head injuries (*Strecker and Ebaugh,* 1924; *Blau,* 1937), behavioural disorders are reported such as lack of motor inhibition, extreme unselectivity in attention, emotional lability, irritability, often without intellectual impairment.

The concept of 'a continuum of degrees of damage' (*Knobloch and Pasamanick,* 1959) led to the view that minor CNS disorders would be likely to manifest themselves in the disorganization of the child's complex behaviour, even in the absence of unequivocal neurological signs. Etiological studies (initially retrospective, later also prospective), indicating relationships between complex behaviour disorders of the MBD type and risk factors early in development, gave some indirect support to this view. Such findings do not justify, however, the 'reversed' reasoning that behaviour disorders in themselves are sufficient evidence for brain damage or brain dysfunction. *Strauss* and associates are generally held responsible for the introduction of this sort of reasoning. They initially identified a number of psychological characteristics distinguishing brain-injured from non-brain-injured mentally retarded children (*Strauss and Kephart,* 1940; *Strauss and Lehtinen,* 1947), whereas they later assume that the presence of such characteristics in themselves indicates brain damage.

These various developments all contributed to the view of 'minimal brain damage' as a primary causative factor in the development of complex learning and/or behaviour disorders in children. Replacement of the term 'minimal brain damage' by 'minimal brain dysfunction' was more an indication of modesty than a contribution to the insight in the problem of neurobehavioural connections in children.

In this respect the Oxford conference in 1962 was important (*Bax and MacKeith,* 1963). Participants agreed that the term 'minimal brain damage' should be abandoned, because of lack of evidence that structural defects formed the basis for the behavioural disorders the group was discussing. No agreement was reached, however, about another term to cover this heterogenous group of children. The editors issued the proceedings of the meeting under the title of 'minimal cerebral dysfunction'. This label together with 'minimal brain dysfunction' replaced the earlier tag of 'minimal brain damage'.

Complications in the Study of MBD

A barrier to further interdisciplinary study is the discrepancy in refinedness and standardization of methods and the different level of abstraction of measures applied in the various disciplines. In medicine a major problem is the assessment and evaluation of slightly deviant neurological functions, for which the term 'soft signs' was introduced.

However, as indicated by *Rutter et al.* (1970) the term 'soft' is most confusing, because it may qualify at least three types of phenomena: (1) Signs of developmental delay in functions such as speech, language, motor co-ordination, perception, etc. (2) Signs due to both neurological and non-neurological factors (nystagmus, strabismus). (3) Slight abnormalities (generally minor examples of classical neurological signs) which are difficult to detect, such as slight asymmetries of tone, etc.

The indication 'soft' may refer to either the inconsistency of the phenomena, the unreliability of their measurement, or to their dubious validity as indicators of the integrity of the CNS.

Furthermore, the study of MBD is complicated by the following factors:

(a) A lack of normative data on the neurological and neurobehavioural development in young children, despite considerable progress in the field of developmental neurology during the last decades. Data have been collected by *Beintema* (1968) over the first 10 days postnatally and by *Touwen* (1976) over the period from birth to walking freely. In older children, only a few scattered data on the distribution of single neurological signs have been reported until now (*Connolly and Stratton,* 1968; *Grant et al.*, 1973).

(b) A lack of precise knowledge of the implications of slight neurological deviations (e.g., with respect to lateralization of functions, intensity of motor reactions, visuo-motor co-ordination, etc.) for the child's behavioural development.

(c) Complex and largely unknown relationships between 'structural' and 'functional' properties of the developing nervous system. The growing CNS has an enormous capacity to compensate functionally for early damage (*Sperry,* 1968), whereas differences in vulnerability of the brain relate to the developmental stage of the organism (*Dobbing and Smart,* 1974).

(d) Early damage due to pre- and perinatal complications usually concerns larger parts of the brain than damage in later life. This is one of the reasons that behavioural disorders are more diversified in children than is to be found in adults. Such lesions are basically of a venous infarctional nature (*Towbin,* 1971). However, cerebral hypoxic lesions have a different character in the premature, affecting primarily the periventricular deposits of germinal tissue, than in the at terms, in which group cell loss mainly concerns the cortex.

(e) In children even more than in adults the behavioural effects of organic disorders are profoundly modified by the environmental conditions (e.g., in lower social economic classes perinatal and early neurological complications seem to have a much stronger effect on children's mental development, than in groups with more favourable environmental conditions) (*Werner et al.,* 1971). An excellent review of the evidence is given by *Sameroff and Chandler* (1975).

(f) Complex relationships between children's behaviour before and after the occurrence of a brain disorder, the precise character of which relationships is generally unknown. Evidently, there exists a category of 'accident prone' children, for whom premorbid data are often unreliable and incomplete (*Bender,* 1956).

Present State of Knowledge

Signs of neurological dysfunction (including EEG abnormalities) are found consistently more often in children presenting learning and/or behaviour disorders of the MBD type than in matched controls (*Schain,* 1970; *Hughes,* 1971; *Werry,* 1972; *Satterfield et al.,* 1971; *Myklebust,* 1973). Children are termed hyperactives, underachievers, MBD cases, etc.; the neurological concomitants include soft signs, unspecified EEG disorders, longer latency and lower amplitude evoked cortical responses, etc. An excellent review of the evidence is given by *Walzer and Richmond* (1973). More signs of neurological dysfunction have also been found in delinquent boys and blind children than in normal children (*Wolff and Hurwitz,* 1966).

In a large number of epidemiological studies complex learning and behaviour disorders of the MBD type have been reported as sequelae of pre- and perinatal complications, such as anoxia and hypoxia (*Rosenfeld and Bradley,* 1948; *Fraser and Wilks,* 1959; *Schachter and Apgar,* 1959; *Knobloch and Pasamanick,* 1966) prematurity or dysmaturity (*Knobloch et al.,* 1956) toxic factors, such as lead poisoning (*Mellins and Jenkins,* 1955) and infective diseases (*Lurie and Levy,* 1942; *Hohman,* 1922), and malnutrition in infancy (*Richardson et al.,* 1973), suggesting a neurological basis for such disorders. However, outcomes of various studies are far from unequivocal, partly due to methodological differences (*Gottfried,* 1973).

To date, one of the few studies, which demonstrated behavioural differences between groups distinguished solely on the basis of neurological dysfunctions, is the study by *Wolff and Hurwitz* (1973). Children in this study presenting choreiform dyskinesia received less favourable behavioural ratings from teachers than nonchoreiforms. *Rutter et al.* (1966) failed to find such associations.

There is a lack of experimental studies, but no shortage of clinical-impressionistic articles in the area of MBD (*Zimet and Fishman,* 1970). This has been extensively discussed in a previous survey (*Kalverboer,* 1971).

Particularly, data are lacking on the later development (into adolescence and adulthood) of children originally suffering from behavioural and learning problems of the MBD type.

By far the best clinical neuropsychiatric study into the significance of brain disorders for behavioural development is that by *Rutter et al.* (1970) reported in 'A Neuropsychiatric Study in Childhood'. However, these authors focus on psychiatric characteristics of children with cerebral palsy, epilepsy, and a number of other unequivocal pathological conditions. They refrain from studying 'the group of less well-defined, borderline neurological disorders', which are just those disorders typically reported in relation to the MBD concept.

As far as objective measurement of behaviour is concerned, one of the best studies is that by *Schulman et al.* (1965) on relationships between behavioural, psycho-metric and neurological measures in a group of 35 retarded boys. They introduce a number of objective measures for the evaluation of behavioural aspects, such as inconsistency, distractibility, hyperactivity and emotional lability. However, they relate their behavioural findings to global ratings of brain damage derived from psychometric tests (WISC), EEGs, and neurological examinations, the validity of which ratings as indicators of brain damage may be seriously doubted. *Schulman* is by no means the worst offender in using subjective and arbitrary measures. Similar usage, employing such terms as 'organicity', 'brain damage', and 'brain dysfunction', can be found in more recent literature (*Sainz,* 1966; *Paine,* 1968; *Wender,* 1971).

Birch (1964) suggests that 'medical and psychological examiners tend to use one another as the essential independent proof of the validity of their inferences'.[1] Written in 1963, this statement still largely holds. Often it is impossible

[1] Many years ago a visitor to a small garrison town was impressed by the fact that each evening, at the stroke of five, the artillery sergeant lowered the colours and ordered his squad to fire a cannon. Amazed at such punctuality, the visitor enquired of the sergeant as to how he determined when it was precisely five o'clock. The sergeant replied that the town was famous not only for the excellence of its garrison but because one of its inhabitants was perhaps the best clock-maker in the world. 'Each morning', he said, 'as I walk past the clock-maker's shop I re-set my own watch and therefore know that when I fire the cannon it is precisely five o'clock'. Only partially satisfied by this answer, the visitor went into town and addressed himself to the clock-maker, saying 'Sir, could you please tell me how you achieved your reputation for having clocks that are always precisely on time?' The clock-maker replied, 'Well, living in this town I have a special advantage. You see, every evening precisely at five o'clock the garrison gun goes off and I re-set all my clocks at that time.'

to obtain a direct and unequivocal proof of brain damage or brain dysfunction. *Birch and Demb* (1953) point out that, as a result, the clinical diagnosis of brain damage in children with adjustment problems is made more often than not, on essentially behavioural grounds.

Benton (1962) argues that many studies, intended to disclose 'state of the organism-response' relationships, only reflect 'response-response' relationships. Although it may be very useful to establish such connections, they do not tell us much about the consequences of brain damage, because an independent criterium for brain damage is lacking.

In the light of the above discussion the best strategy in MBD studies in children seems to be to analyze in detail the behavioural repertoire in relevant situations and to relate findings to those obtained in comprehensive neurological assessments. This was attempted in an observational study of our own on 150 preschool children, born in the University Hospital in Groningen, in which study focus was on a core problem in the MBD case: the implications of a non-optimal neurological condition for the child's free-field activity (*Kalverboer,* 1975). Although the MBD label could not be applied to most children in this study, findings may throw some light on the usefulness of the MBD concept.

There are two major contrasts with previous MBD work: (a) preschool-aged children were studied, not selected on the basis of referrals, and (b) 'objective' assessments of the child's free-field behaviour were related to standardized neurological assessments, according to the method described by *Touwen and Prechtl* (1970).

Categories were developed for the description of motor, visual and verbal aspects of the behaviour that allowed for a detailed analysis of the child's exploration of the room, contact with the mother, play behaviour, waiting behaviour, etc. (data from video-recordings and direct observations). A detailed analysis of the 'structure' of the behavioural repertoire preceded the search for neurobehavioural relationships.

Main conclusions from the results of this study were the following:

(a) Neurobehavioural relationships are found in all observational conditions. However (1) they are too low for any prediction about individuals, and (2) they strongly depend on the situation in which behaviour is observed.

(b) Intra- and inter-individual variability of behaviour is the main finding: general labels, such as 'hyperactivity' and MBD, are useless as indices of children's problem behaviour.

(c) There are clear-cut sex differences in behaviour *per se* and in neurobehavioural relationships: MBD may mean something different for boys and girls (dysfunction vs. dysmaturity).

(d) Children with minor neurological dysfunctions may function quite well in appropriate environments: 'handicaps' seem to relate to a lack of sustained attention in non-stimulating situations.

(e) The term 'soft neurological signs' underestimates the differentiated relationships between minor neurological dysfunctions (e.g. choreiform dyskinesia) and behaviour. An approach of relating such 'soft' signs to complex clinical phenomena is fruitless.

Conclusions

What conclusions can be drawn from a study of the data available up till now?

Terms such as MBD (minimal brain dysfunction) and SLD (special learning disorders) refer to a group of children heterogeneous with respect to the disorders they present and the possible etiology of their adaptational problems.

Gomez (1967) considered the introduction of a diagnostic label such as 'minimal cerebral dysfunction' as a backward step in the nosology of disorders of behaviour and learning, and pleaded for more descriptive sub-classifications. He argued for refraining from the use of such labels in an article entitled 'Minimum Cerebral Dysfunction, Maximum Neurological Confusion'.

Some people have suggested using more descriptive terms, such as 'delayed or irregular maturation' (*Abrams,* 1968). However, as stated by *Dinnage* (1970), 'whatever term is used, it refers to a mixed group of handicaps with no known organic basis'.

There is no scientific evidence linking behavioural disorders and independent signs of neurological dysfunction in children which would justify including them all in one 'minimal brain dysfunction syndrome' (*Schulman et al.*, 1965; *Rutter et al.*, 1966; *Werry,* 1968). Until yet EEG data have not given a real contribution to our understanding of the syndrome: the most common finding is 'diffuse generalized abnormality of the EEG' or 'borderline EEG'. So-called 'biochemical theories' about the background of the MBD problems – as given, for example, by *Wender* (1971) – seem to be mere speculations on the basis of animal data of dubious relevance for the MBD problem. Even the relationships among the behavioural features themselves may be much weaker than is generally assumed (*Routh and Roberts,* 1972). Often such relationships depend more on the perceptual and cognitive schemata of the observer than on the factual behaviour of the child.

Further study of neurobehavioural relationships is needed to achieve a better understanding of the MBD problem. Both neurological and behavioural assessments are to a considerable extent concerned with behavioural functions or performances of the child. How such performances are related to structural properties of the brain or to brain processes is largely unknown. This should be considered when talking about 'neurobehavioural' relationships. On the one hand, difficulties in both areas may be manifestations of some underlying (neurological) disorder affecting the functional organization in all its facets: on the other hand difficulties in the behavioural area may be a secondary effect of minor neurological dysfunctions, e.g., the presence of neurological dysfunction such as dyskinesia may prevent the child from performing complex activities smoothly and efficiently, such as writing, building with blocks, etc.

It is a fair estimation that approximately 10% of school-aged children develop learning and/or behavioural disorders, which in one way or another relate to their neurological condition. Further systematic and close follow-up studies, starting early in development, and taking into account the intimate interaction between biological and environmental (social and physical) factors in the determination of developmental disorders, will be necessary to detect more precisely the background of their problems. Such knowledge is essential for the development of adequate educational and didactical procedures. The use of labels, such as MBD or hyperactivity will not be of much help in this respect. Such labels represent to a large extent the biases of the environment towards children with learning and/or behavioural problems and are in many instances artefacts of our instruments and statistical techniques.

We may end with the paradoxical conclusion put forward by *Dinnage* (1970): 'While there is no evidence that the minimally brain-damaged child exists, he urgently needs our attention.'

Summary

The wide interest in the MBD problem is traced back to converging developments in education, psychology, and medical thinking during the last half century. Child-centred didactical methods and the development of specific approaches for children with limitations in their learning abilities went parallel to a rapid development of refined psychodiagnostic tools and basic theoretical insights on connections between somatic and mental aspects of the development. In neuropsychology the CNS became considered as an integrated, differentiated system, in which diffuse damage would lead to general deficits in the behavioural organization. Further, findings in relation to aphasia in adults and sequelae of brain damage in children together with the idea of a continuum of the degrees of damage led to the conception of a neurological background for adaptational problems in children.

Despite this widespread interest, it is pointed out that progress in the study of MBD was slow. This is attributed partly to differences in refinement and standardization of methods in the different disciplines, partly to complicated relationships between neurological condition and behaviour in early phases of development. Many studies show fallacies and these are briefly indicated.

Some data are presented from an observational study on neurobehavioural relationships in preschool children. Meaningful relationships between neurology and behaviour were found in all observational conditions. However, intra- and inter-individual variability was the main finding. Findings point to the complex determination of behavioural differences and suggest that linking any behaviour directly to an implication of brain damage is dangerous. General labels such as MBD or hyperactivity should be avoided.

References

Abrams, A.L.: Delayed and irregular maturation versus minimal brain injury. Clin. Pediat. *7:* 344 (1968).

Bax, M. and MacKeith, R.: Minimal cerebral dysfunction. Little Club Clinics in Developmental Medicine, No. 10 (Heinemann, London 1963).

Beach, F.A.; Hebb, D.O.; Morgan, C.G., and Nissen, H.W.: The neuropsychology of Lashley (McGraw-Hill, New York 1960).

Beintema, D.J.: A neurological study of newborn infants. Little Club Clinics in Developmental Medicine, No. 28 (Heinemann, London 1968).

Bender, L.: Psychopathology of children with organic brain disorders, part III–IV (Thomas, Springfield 1956).

Benton, A.L.: Behavioural indices of brain injury in school children. Child Dev. *33:* 199 (1962).

Birch, H.G.: Brain damage in children (Williams & Wilkins, Baltimore 1964).

Birch, H.G. and Demb, H.: The information and extinction of conditional reflexes in 'brain-damaged' and mongoloid children. J. nerv. ment. Dis. *129:* 162 (1953).

Blau, A.: Mental changes following head trauma in children. Archs Neurol. Psychiat. *35:* 722–769 (1937).

Bond, E.D.: Postencephalitic, ordinary and extraordinary children. J. Pediat. *1:* 310–314 (1932).

Boring, E.G.: Lashley and cortical integration; in *Beach, Hebb, Morgan and Nissen* The neuropsychology of Lashley (McGraw-Hill, New York 1960).

Connolly, K. and Stratton, P.: Developmental changes in associated movements. Dev. Med. Child Neurol. *10:* 49–56 (1968).

Dinnage, R.: The handicapped child. Studies in child development: research review, vol. 1 (Longman, London 1970).

Dobbing, J. and Smart, J.L.: Vulnerability of developing brain and behaviour. Br. med. Bull. *19:* 164–168 (1974).

Fraser, M.S. and Wilks, J.: The residual effects of neonatal asphyxia. J. Obstet. Gynaec. Br. Empire *66:* 748 (1959).

Gomez, M.R.: Minimal cerebral dysfunction (maximal neurological confusion). Clin. Pediat. *6:* 589 (1967).

Gottfried, A.W.: Intellectual consequences of perinatal anoxia. Psychol. Bull. *80:* 232 (1973).

Grant, W.W.; Boelsche, A.N., and Zin, D.: Developmental patterns of two motor functions. Dev. Med. Child Neurol. *15:* 171 (1973).

Hohman, L.B.: Post-encephalitic behavior disorders. Johns Hopkins Hosp. Bull. *33:* 372–375 (1922).

Hughes, J.: Electroencephalography and learning disabilities; in *Myklebust* Progress in learning disabilities, vol. 2 (Grune & Stratton, New York 1971).

Kalverboer, A.F.: Over de relatie tussen neurologische dysfuncties en gedrag bij kinderen; in *De Wit, Bolle and Jessurun Cardozo-van Hoorn* Psychologen over het kind (Wolters-Noordhoff, Groningen 1971).

Kalverboer, A.E.: A neurobehavioural study in preschool children. Clinics in developmental medicine, No. 54 (SIMP/Heinemann, London 1975).

Knobloch, H. and Pasamanick, B.: Syndrome of minimal damage in infancy. J. Am. med. Ass. *170:* 1384–1387 (1959).

Knobloch, H. and Pasamanick, B.: Prospective studies on the epidemiology of reproductive casualty. Methods, findings and some implications. Merrill-Palmer Q. *12:* 27 (1966).

Knobloch, H.; Rider, R.; Harper, P., and Pasamanick, B.: Neuropsychiatric sequelae of prematurity. J. Am. med. Ass. *161:* 581 (1956).

Lashley, K.S.: Basic neural mechanisms in behavior. Psychol. Rev. *37:* 1–24 (1930).

Lashley, K.S.: In search of the engram. Symp. Soc. exp. Biol. *4:* 454 (1950).

Lashley, K.S.: The problem of serial order in behavior; in *Jeffress* Cerebral mechanisms in behavior. The Hixon symposium (Wiley, New York 1951).

Lashley, K.S.: Cerebral organization and behavior; in The brain and human behavior. Proc. Ass. Res. nerv. ment. Dis. *36:* 1 (1958).

Luria A.R.: The working brain (Penguin Books, Harmondsworth 1973).

Lurie, L.A. and Levy, S.: Behavior disorders – personality changes and behavior disorders of children following pertussis. J. Am. med. Ass. *120B:* 890–894 (1942).

Mellins, R.B. and Jenkins, C.D.: Epidemiological and psychological study of lead poisoning in children. J. Am. med. Ass. *158:* 15 (1955).

Myklebust, H.R.: Identification and diagnosis of children with learning disabilities: an interdisciplinary study of criteria. Semin. Psychiat. *5:* 55 (1973).

Paine, R.: Syndromes of 'minimal cerebral damage'. Pediat. Clins N. Am. *15:* 779 (1968).

Richardson, S.A.; Birch, H.G., and Hertzig, M.E.: School performance of children who were severely malnourished in infancy. Am. J. ment. Defic. *77:* 623 (1973).

Rosenfeld, G.B. and Bradley, C.: Childhood behavior sequelae of asphyxia in infancy with special reference to pertussis and asphyxia neonatorum. Pediatrics, Springfield *2:* 74.

Routh, D.K. and Roberts, R.D.: Minimal brain dysfunction in children. Failure to find evidence for a behavioral syndrome. Psychol. Rep. *31:* 307 (1972).

Rutter, M.; Graham, P., and Birch, H.G.: Interrelations between the choreiform syndrome, reading disability and psychiatric disorder in children of 8–11. Devl Med. Child Neurol. *8:* 149 (1966).

Rutter, M.; Graham, P., and Yule, W.: A neuropsychiatric study in childhood. Clinics in developmental medicine, No. 35/36 (SIMP/Heinemann, London 1970).

Sameroff, A.J. and Chandler, M.J.: Reproductive risk and the continuum of caretaking casualty; in *Horowitz, Hetherington, Scarr-Salapatek and Siegel* Review of child developmental research, vol. 4 (University of Chicago Press, Chicago 1975).

Satterfield, J.H. and Dawson, M.E.: Electrodermal correlates of hyperactivity in children. Psychophysiology *8:* 191 (1971).

Schachter, F.F. and Apgar, V.: Perinatal asphyxia and psychological signs of brain damage in childhood. Pediatrics, Springfield *24:* 1016 (1959).

Schain, R.J.: Neurological evaluation of children with learning disorders. Neuropädiatrie *1:* 307 (1970).

Schulman, J.L.; Kaspar, J.C., and Throne, F.M.: Brain damage and behavior. A clinical-experimental study (Thomas, Springfield 1965).

Sperry, R.W.: Plasticity of neural maturation. Devl Biol., suppl. 2, p. 306 (1968).

Strauss, A.A. and Kephart, N.C.: Behavior differences in mentally retarded children measured by a new behavior rating scale. Am. J. Psychiat. *96:* 1117 (1940).

Strauss, A.A. and Lehtinen, L.E.: Psychopathology and education of the brain-injured child, vol. 1 (Grune & Stratton, New York 1947).

Strecker, E.A. and Ebaugh, F.G.: Neuropsychiatric sequelae of cerebral trauma in children. Archs Neurol. Psychiat. *12:* 443 (1924).

Strother, C.R.: Minimal cerebral dysfunction. A historical overview; in *De la Cruz, Fox, Roberts and Tarjan* Minimal brain dysfunction. Ann. N.Y. Acad. Sci. *205* (1973).

Touwen, B.C.L.: Neurological development in infancy. Clinics in developmental medicine, No. 58 (SIMP/Heinemann, London 1976).

Touwen, B.C.L. and Prechtl, H.F.R.: The neurological examination of the child with minor nervous dysfunction. Clinics in developmental medicine, No. 38 (SIMP/Heinemann, London 1970).

Walzer, S. and Richmond, J.B.: The epidemiology of learning disorders. Pediat. Clin N. Am. *20:* 549 (1973).

Wedell, K.: Learning and perceptuo-motor disabilities in children (Wiley, London 1973).

Wender, P.H.: Minimal brain dysfunction in children (Wiley-Interscience, New York 1971).

Werner, E.E.; Bierman, J.M., and French, F.E.: The children of Kauai (University of Hawaii, Honolulu 1971).

Werry, J.S.: Studies on the hyperactive child. IV. An empirical analysis of the minimal brain dysfunction syndrome. Archs gen. Psychiat. *19:* 9 (1968).

Werry, J.S.: Organic factors in childhood psychopathology; in *Quay and Werry* Psychopathological disorders in childhood (Wiley, New York 1972).

Wolff, P.H. and Hurwitz, I.: The choreiform syndrome. Devl Med. Child Neurol. *8:* 160 (1966).

Wolff, P.H. and Hurwitz, I.: Functional implications of the minimal brain damage syndrome; in *Walzer and Wolff* Minimal cerebral dysfunction in children. Semin. Psychiat. *5:* 105 (1973).

Zimet, C.N. and Fishman, D.B.: Psychological deficit in schizophrenia and brain damage. Ann. Rev. Psychol. *21:* 113 (1970).

Dr. *A.F. Kalverboer,* Laboratory for Experimental Clinical Psychology,
Dept. of Clinical Psychology, State University Groningen, Turfsingel 46,
Groningen (The Netherlands)

Adv. biol. Psychiat., vol. 1, pp. 18–34 (Karger, Basel 1978)

Longitudinal Research and the Minimal Brain Damage Syndrome

D. Shaffer

Division of Child Psychiatry, Department of Psychiatry, New York Psychiatric Institute, New York, N.Y.

Introduction

Minimal brain damage (MBD) is an unsatisfactory diagnosis. Its existence is questioned by many, others who accept and use it, do so in very different ways and, despite claims to the contrary, little is known of its aetiology or treatment. Few would disagree with the by-now familiar criticisms that are heard – complex and highly speculative notions about mechanisms and aetiology, the apparent heterogeneity and non-specificity of its manifestations, and not least its ambiguous title – all of which make it an easy target. However, in making these criticisms it is clearly important not to throw the baby out with the bathwater. Rather what is needed is a constructive and analytical approach to sort out useful from irrelevant aspects of this concept.

The study of the natural history of a condition is an important part of this process of *concept* definition and validation. Strong support for the existence of the syndrome would be brought if it could be shown that children with a given constellation of clinical features shared a common outcome, and differed in this from children who lacked its necessary components. Furthermore, it is in its power to predict outcome that the familiar medical model – to which the concept of a syndrome belongs – has its greatest strength.

However, the uncertainty which surrounds the concept of the MBD syndrome makes its study no easy task. The MBD syndrome is most comprehensively used to describe behaviour difficulties (in particular hyperactivity and inattention) along with academic underachievement, a history of earlier physical stress, such as perinatal complication or head injury and, on examination, a variety of non-localising neurological signs and poor or uneven performance on a variety of measures of intelligence and perceptual and motor function. Yet very few workers or clinicians have insisted that all these features be present nor have they distinguished between children with some but not other features and the literature abounds with descriptive treatment and a small number of follow-up studies in which the diagnosis has been made with a variable number of criteria.

A further complication is that follow-up studies require time. The adults and adolescents that are being written about today were first seen between 10 and 20 years ago, often by clinicians who were not sensitised to the notions of the *'hyperkinetic syndrome'* or 'minimal brain damage syndrome', nor to the problems associated with these terms. These studies may depend on retrospective case note examinations and may lack appropriate controls.

Because of these limitations, I intend to approach this review by looking separately at studies which have examined the sequelae of 4 of the components of the syndrome, i.e. (i) a history of perinatal complication; (ii) early acute disturbances of the CNS, i.e. infection, trauma, or metabolic upset; (iii) the presence of soft neurological signs, and (iv) so-called hyperkinetic behaviour disorder. Outcome variables that are being examined are psychiatric state, social adjustment, educational achievement, and intelligence. It is well to bear in mind that all of these are overwhelmingly influenced by environmental factors such as emotional support within the family and levels of educational stimulation and that any credible investigation will have needed to take these into account.

Sequelae of Perinatal Difficulties

The clinician is often influenced in making a diagnosis of MBD by a history of perinatal difficulties which although not resulting in enduring neurological damage – detectable by the usual clinical methods – is considered to have been a factor in the development of the patient's learning or behaviour disorder. To what extent do such assumptions receive support from follow-up studies?

A history of abnormal gestation or delivery, low birth weight and neonatal asphyxia is common among children attending psychiatric clinics. It is largely as a consequence of such observations (*Knobloch and Pasamanick,* 1966) that emphasis on the neurological basis of disturbed behaviour in childhood has acquired such acceptance. However, before concluding that minor degrees of brain damage suffered during the peri-natal period have a causal relationship with later learning and behaviour problems, two considerations should be borne in mind:

(a) Perinatal abnormality is not independent of social and family disadvantage – at least in the United Kingdom and in many communities in the United States. Thus, *Chamberlain et al.* (1976) in their survey of all births taking place in the United Kingdom during a given week in 1970, noted a close correlation between *perinatal mortality* and maternal height, which was in turn strongly related to *social class.* Similarly, perinatal mortality among illegitimate births is approximately twice the national average and it is also increased in births to widowed, divorced and separated mothers, to mothers under the age of 16 and to the late born children of large families (*Butler and Alberman,* 1969). *Birth weight* too is directly related to social class and such seemingly biological phenomena as neo-natal convulsions are rare in breast-fed children and possibly as a consequence, were found by *Chamberlain* to occur significantly less often among middle class mothers. These correlations are all likely to increase an apparent relationship between perinatal hazard and later intellectual deficit or behavioural problems, which might in reality be more a consequence of the disadvantageous environment in which the child has been reared. Artefacts of this sort can only be identified by studies in which a comparison is made between groups with comparable degrees of disadvantage, educational opportunity and stimulation, etc. Simple matching for parental occupation will rarely suffice.

(b) *Perinatal complications* are common. In *Chamberlain*'s survey it was found that approximately 5% of all infants took longer than 3 min to establish regular respiration and as many as 11% spent some time during their 1st week of life in a special care unit. Yet by no means all of these children will have suffered from brain damage. The management given to a new-born infant may be influenced as much by the available resources as by need. As used clinically, the term perinatal complications may encompass either unusual management, e.g., having been in a special care unit or a complication affecting the process of gestation or delivery which did not necessarily affect the well being of the fetus, e.g., forceps delivery, as well as illness in the infant. 'Peri-natal complications' are therefore an imperfect index of brain injury. Follow-up studies which start from such a crude index are likely to obscure relationships between early brain damage and later outcome by the inclusion of many cases in which brain damage did not take place. It seems likely that follow-up studies which start with a more direct index of neonatal neurological state (*Prechtl,* 1965) will have a better chance of demonstrating an antecedent causal relationship.

Given these difficulties what evidence is there that *perinatal illness* increases the likelihood of later psychiatric disorder or reduced IQ? Ideally, any follow-up investigation would take *neo-natal neurological state,* rather than perinatal complication as a starting point and would take full account of home care and stimulation. No such study has yet been carried out. However, *Kalverboer et al.* (1973) re-examined, at the age of 5, 33 children without gross brain damage who had shown non-localising neurological abnormalities when examined during the neonatal period. No relationship was noted between the initial and later neurological state and there was only a weak relationship with behaviour measured in an experimental situation. Children who had suffered from the neonatal *'apathy syndrome'* (*Prechtl,* 1965) showed more distress when separated from their mother, and children with the neonatal *'hyperexcitability syndrome'* played *more* constructively under difficult conditions. Social and family factors were uncontrolled, numbers were small and behaviour in an experimental situation may not be representative of behaviour in more complex real life situations. Furthermore – by design – this study excluded more severe forms of neonatal neurological impairment. Nevertheless, further research of this sort, using direct indices of early neurological function, may offer the best opportunity for improving our understanding of relationships between illness *in utero* or infancy and later socio-psychological difficulties. The evidence from adequately controlled studies which have used less direct indicators of initial brain injury varies according to whether behaviour, intelligence or educational achievement is examined.

Behaviour

Werner et al.'s (1968) prospective study of a total population of births on Kuai Island in Hawaii is of particular interest. In this population there was no social class bias with respect to peri-natal complications. Measures of parental IQ and detailed and standardised assessments of home stimulation and emotional support were undertaken during the course of follow-up. Evaluation at age 10 failed to show any relationship between *peri-natal factors* and *later emotional disorder.*

Similarly, *Davie et al.* (1972) reporting on the National Child Development Study, which included all children born in the UK during 1 week in 1958, found only trivial differences in social adjustment between children of normal and low *birth weight* at age 7, after social class had been taken into account. *Graham et al.* (1962) could find no differences in behaviour, at the age of 3, between 350 children who had suffered from clearly documented neonatal asphyxia and a group of carefully matched controls.

Other smaller, less well-controlled investigations have examined behavioural outcome in a detail that is not possible in the larger studies. An interesting example is the University of London longitudinal study reported on by *Ucko* (1965). In this it was noted that previously asphyxiated children were more irregular in *sleeping* and other behaviours, and were generally more difficult to manage than non-asphyxiated children. *Temperamental* differences of this sort, normal in themselves, may nevertheless increase a child's susceptibility to environmental disadvantage.

All in all, however, research does not support the notion that perinatal illness has an independent effect on later behaviour problems, although there may be persisting effects on behavioural style or temperament which are difficult to elicit in large scale studies using relatively crude measures. All studies which take a mixture of *perinatal abnormalities* as a starting point suffer by being inevitably composed of brain-damaged and normal children.

Intelligence

There have been a large number of studies which have examined the relationship between neo-natal asphyxia and other perinatal stress and later intellectual deficit. These have been reviewed by *Gottfried* (1973) and are remarkable for the fact that studies which show such an effect are almost equally balanced by studies which do not.

It seems likely that this is a consequence of imperfect or inadequate control for social and environmental factors. Thus in the Kuai follow-up, initial analysis suggested that at age 10, significantly more of the children with an IQ below 85 had experienced severe *perinatal complications.* However, when the effects of home stimulation and socio-economic class were partialled out there was no residual effect. Similarly, *Fisch et al.* (1976) were able to draw upon the very large population in the United States Collaborative Study, and after carefully controlling on a number of indices of socio-economic and educational status found no relationship between 1- and 5-min Apgar scores and IQ at age 7.

Learning Difficulties

Davie et al. (1972) analysing reading attainment at the age of 7 of children included in the National Child Development Study found a slight but significant relationship between birth weight and later reading attainment after allowing for social class. However, *Werner* using very much more detailed indices of home stimulation, but a somewhat less satisfactory measure of reading attainment, found that the apparent effect of perinatal disorder on reading ability could be accounted for by differences in levels of educational stimulation and emotional support.

Summary

Broadly speaking it is the big follow-up studies – with large numbers of subjects – which can take adequate account of socio-environmental differences. These have failed to show an independent relationship between the early experience of medical difficulties in the peri-natal period and later emotional disturbance, learning difficulties or intellectual backwardness. However, there have also been smaller more-detailed studies which have used subtler measures of assessment and these indicate that early CNS disturbance may lead to differences in temperament, which although not in themselves 'abnormal', may nevertheless increase liability to later disturbance. Furthermore, the negative results of the big studies must be interpreted with caution for none have started with any direct measure of early neurological dysfunction, nor have they attempted to define outcome in terms of those characteristics which are usually held to constitute the MBD syndrome.

Early Acute Disturbances of the CNS

In the previous section I have examined the sequelae of events which are only irregularly associated with brain damage. There are in addition a number of acute conditions affecting the CNS such as infection, trauma and metabolic upset which, if mild, may leave the patient with no enduring abnormality that would be detected on a conventional neurological examination. However, a history of this type of illness may be considered relevant to later behaviour disorder or learning difficulty and is probably influential in making a diagnosis of MBD.

CNS Infection

Children who recover from viral or pyogenic meningitis seem no more likely than noninfected children to develop significant behaviour disturbances, although it must be emphasised that outcome measures and controls in most studies are deficient (*Muller et al.*, 1958; *Gibbs et al.*, 1964). The effects on intelligence are less clear cut – thus, *Dodge and Swartz* (1965), examining mainly older children, found that a history of pyogenic meningitis had no effect on IQ. By contrast, *Sells et al.* (1975) found impairment of IQ and language skills of children who had had an enteroviral infection of the CNS before the age of one. No adverse effects seemed to follow infection at a later age.

Head Injury

Head injury is common in childhood and is a frequent cause for hospital admission. Most injuries are trivial and admission is undertaken to ensure that any late complications are promptly observed. Investigating the later behaviour or achievements of this group – in whom it can reasonably be assumed that some minor degree of brain damage *has* taken place – would be of special interest. If it could be shown that these children ran an increased risk for later psychiatric disorder, support would be given to the notion that slight brain damage could become manifest in cognitive and behavioural disorder, in the absence of persistent motor or sensory abnormality.

However, longitudinal studies of head injury require careful control for there is evidence that children who become involved in accidents differ in their personality (*Mannheimer and Mellinger,* 1967) and are more likely to have behaviour problems before their injury (*Craft,* 1972) than children who do not have accidents. Similarly, it seems likely that there is an excess of family stress in the homes of injured children – for deficiencies in care and supervision at home will increase the chances of exposure to situations in which accidents are likely to occur.

Specific studies on the sequelae of mild *head injury* are lacking but it is clear that psychiatric disorder may follow injury in the absence of persisting motor or sensory signs. An example is *Shaffer et al.*'s (1975) follow-up study in which it was found that almost two-thirds of a head-injured group were disturbed, but that fewer than 10% had any residual neurological impairment. Other studies (*Black et al.,* 1969; *Hjern and Nylander,* 1964; *Klonoff and Paris,* 1974) similarly suggest that psychiatric problems may result from head injury without other clinical evidence of persistent brain damage.

Metabolic Upset

Investigations to study the damage that might be caused to the developing CNS by acute or chronic malnutrition in early childhood (*Cravioto and Delcardie,* 1972) suggest that it is the compounding of *malnutrition* with other forms of social deprivation which result in the poor cognitive and social development of these children. Strategies have therefore been devised to study children from otherwise normal backgrounds in whom malnutrition has resulted from some medical condition. *Ellis and Hill* (1975) contrasted the development of children with cystic fibrosis with and without a history of acute *malnutrition* during infancy. They failed to find an effect on either intelligence or educational development. *Klein et al.* (1975) examined IQ, educational attainment and classroom behaviour in school age children who had suffered from pyloric stenosis with varying degrees of weight loss. They used sibling and non-sibling controls and found that where weight loss had exceeded 10% of body weight there was later impairment of learning ability and, in particular, impairment of short-term memory. Classroom behaviour and social maturity were unaffected.

Another common form of metabolic disturbance which may affect the central nervous system is that associated with high serum *lead* levels. However, high lead levels are found especially often in children with a history of *pica* and in children who live in old and dilapidated accommodation. There are therefore major methodological difficulties in sorting out the effects of pre-existing disorder and social disadvantage. Even such studies as those of *de la Burde and Choate* (1972, 1975) which found significant psychiatric and cognitive effects after very careful and extensive matching of social and family factors, cannot be accepted without question as the high *lead* children still differed with respect to earlier pica and quality of housing. *Lansdown et al.*'s (1974) investigation within a whole community that had been exposed to atmospheric lead pollution suggests a way of overcoming these difficulties. Behaviour ratings and psychological test results were obtained in a total population of 6- to 17-year-olds living near a lead smelter. The children living nearest the smelter were found to have the highest serum lead levels, but no relationship was found between lead and either IQ or behaviour ratings. However, the study may have been confounded by social factors, for the families living closest to the smelter were also more settled, and this may have led to a paradoxical weighting of favourable social factors in favour of the lead exposed group.

Summary

In contrast with perinatal complications – which as mentioned above are imperfect indicators that the child has sustained injury to the CNS – there is some evidence that a history of mild head injury or metabolic upset may lead to later cognitive or behavioural difficulties in the absence of persisting motor and sensory handicaps. However, the effects are not strong and the methods used to study them leave room for doubts.

Minor Neurological Signs and Psychiatric Disorder in Adolescence and Adult Life

A number of neurological signs have been described as occurring more frequently in groups of children with behaviour or learning problems than in 'normal' children (*Adams et al.*, 1974; *Kennard*, 1960; *Rutter et al.*, 1966; *Stine et al.*, 1975; *Wolff and Hurwitz*, 1973). Such signs include involuntary movements of a choreic or athetoid type, motor abnormalities such as synkinesis (mirror movements), dysdiadochokinesis (difficulty in performing rapid alternating movements) and general clumsiness as well as sensory abnormalities, in particular dysgraphaesthesia (inability to identify or reproduce shapes outlined by the examiner on the palmar surface of the child's outstretched hand).

Such signs are often referred to as being *'soft'*. *Rutter et al.* (1970a) have pointed out that the term 'soft' is used to describe different groups of signs for quite different reasons. Some are labelled 'soft' because they run a developmental course and do not have any clear locus of origin. Such signs are not pointers to disease in the traditional sense and their pathological roots are obscure. Most of the signs mentioned above, all of which are age-related (*Peters et al.*, 1975), would come into this category. Most, however, can be elicited readily and reliably (*Rutter et al.*, 1970a). A different group of signs are considered 'soft' because they are minor in degree and because they are difficult to detect in a reliable fashion. Such signs would include reflex or tone asymmetries.

Soft signs occur in many otherwise normal children. Thus, *Adams et al.* (1974) found that 10% of 9- to 11-year-olds without behaviour or learning problems had dysgraphaesthesia and 8% dysdiadochokinesis. *Rutter et al.* (1970a) found that 14% of normal 10- to 11-year-olds showed mirror movements and *Wolff and Hurwitz* (1966) found that choreatiform movements could be elicited in 11% of normal children.

Almost all studies have shown a relationship between the presence of these signs and age and IQ. They are also sex related, and for a given age and IQ occur more frequently in boys. When such factors are taken into account many signs fail to discriminate between problem and nonproblem children, although both *dysdiadochokinesis* and *dysgraphaesthesia* are found more often in disturbed children even after taking account of age, sex and IQ (*Adams et al.*, 1974; *Myklebust*, 1973; *Peters et al.*, 1975).

We do not know whether the association with disorder is increased if such signs persist into adolescence or adulthood. However, a number of studies have appeared over the past decade which suggest that they are found especially often in older patients suffering from particular types of psychiatric disturbance. The studies have been such that it is not possible to tell whether the soft signs have been present since childhood, nor is it possible to determine what – if any – type of disorder would have been diagnosable during childhood.

The association was first noted by *Hertzig and Birch* (1966, 1968) who examined successive cases admitted to the adolescent service at Bellevue Hospital. A high proportion of *psychotic* patients were found to have abnormal *soft signs.* However, these studies were uncontrolled, did not take account of current drug intake and included some patients with frank neurological disease. *Rochford et al.* (1970) examined 65 random admissions to 3 adult psychiatric units. Examination took place after a drug-free period of 48 h and 20 staff controls were studies as well. This study found an excess of soft signs among *schizophrenic* patients and patients diagnosed as having a personality disorder, but no excess in patients with an affective illness. It is questionable whether the drug-free period was of sufficient length and the use of staff controls would have rendered the study non-blind.

Mosher et al. (1971) have undertaken a clinical neurological examination on 15 pairs of identical twins discordant for *schizophrenia.* 11 out of 15 of the discordant twins had *abnormal signs* compared with 3 out of 15 of the unaffected siblings. The authors are cautious about drawing conclusions from this study for the probands differed with respect to previous intake of phenothiazine drugs, ECT and hospitalisation. Nor can this study indicate whether abnormal findings are specific for schizophrenia. In most twin studies there is an excess of perinatal abnormality and so no conclusions about the prevalence of signs amongst schizophrenics can be drawn.

In many respects the most satisfactory investigation has been that by *Quitkin et al.* (1976). Earlier studies had suggested to these workers that adult schizophrenics who had experienced marked personality difficulties in childhood (characteristically being friendless, having academic difficulties and narrow interests) were especially likely to have a neurological abnormality for they often gave a history of delayed developmental milestones, learning problems at school and had uneven score patterns on psychometric examination. They labelled this group schizophrenia with premorbid asociality (SPA). For similar reasons they suspected an organic basis in certain patients with a *personality disorder.* These were patients who were characteristically antisocially impulsive and who had frequent but brief non-reactive mood swings. They have called this group emotionally unstable character disorder (EUCD). In the study under discussion they examined 298 consecutive admissions under the age of 50 none of whom had organic neurological disease or had been treated previously with ECT. All patients were withdrawn from drugs for at least 10 days before examination. The reliability and consistency of the examination was systematically assessed and was carried out blind to the psychiatric rating. Both the SPA and the EUCD groups differed from other diagnostic categories in more commonly exhibiting dysdiadochokinesis, agraphaesthesia, mirror movements, finger apraxia and disturbances of speech and gait. There was no excess of such signs in patients with other forms of schizophrenia, affective disorder or other types of personality disorder. The importance of a drug-free period was emphasised by a subsidiary finding of a high prevalence of signs in a group of diagnostically mixed patients receiving drugs.

These studies suggest, but do not confirm, the proposition that disturbed children with neurological dysfunction are predisposed to develop fairly specific psychiatric syndromes in adult life. Before drawing such conclusions it will be necessary to examine the correlates of *soft signs* in an unselected adult population, a study which has yet to be carried out. These studies also point to the value of distinguishing between disturbed children with neurological dysfunction and those without, in clinical follow-up studies.

Follow-Up Studies of the Hyperkinetic Syndrome

Strauss and Lehtinen (1947), *Clements and Peters* (1962) and other exponents of the minimal brain dysfunction syndrome at one time held that brain injury could be inferred by characteristic behaviour disturbance and, in particular, by hyperactivity, even in the absence of other evidence of neurological disorder. To some extent psychiatrists such as *Wender* (1972) have moved away from this position, suggesting that almost all forms of disturbance in childhood may be a manifestation of underlying brain dysfunction. Although there is little to support *Wender*'s suggestions that brain dysfunction underlies most psychiatric disturbance in childhood, the change from beliefs in pathognomonic syndromes is welcome as being more in accordance with available facts.

Brain-injured children are susceptible to all types of psychiatric disorder, and there is no good evidence that they are especially likely to develop any particular one. This was shown in the Isle of Wight survey (*Rutter et al.,* 1970a) of all children with a CNS or epileptic disorder, where the range of diagnoses amongst affected children with a disturbance was broadly similar to that found amongst non-brain-injured children. However, surveys of this sort may fail to show relationships between some uncommon psychiatric conditions occurring predominantly or uniquely amongst children with brain pathology. An example of this sort might be the hyperkinetic syndrome which although diagnosed frequently in North America is made sparingly in Europe.

Very few children were diagnosed as *hyperactive* in the Isle of Wight survey, but the syndrome did occur slightly, but not significantly, more often amongst children with brain damage.

The diagnosis was only used in that study when the child was reported to be overactive by both parents and teacher, was overactive on examination by the psychiatrist and when there was no evidence of any other type of psychiatric disorder. However, the diagnosis as commonly used in the USA is unsatisfactory being both imprecise and unreliable. One reason for this is that in practice it appears to rely heavily on parents or teachers reports of overactivity or poor concentration. Yet these descriptions seem to be used with little discrimination. For example, *Lapouse and Monk* (1958) noted that more than 50% of parents in an unselected population considered their son to be overactive. Similarly, in the Isle of Wight Survey (*Rutter et al.*, 1960b) one-third of 10- to 11-year-old boys who were ultimately judged not to have a psychiatric disorder were described as overactive or inattentive by both parents and teachers.

Given that reports of overactivity are not in themselves a reliable indicator of psychiatric disorder, is there evidence that activity level, when measured objectively, relates in any way to brain damage? *Schulman et al.* (1965) compared the whole day motor activities of brain-damaged children with controls using an actometer device and found no difference. *Werry et al.* (1972) refer to a number of factor analytic studies which show little tendency for *hyperactivity,* inattention, emotional lability or inconsistency to relate, either to each other or to indices of brain damage. However, it might be that brain-damaged children are more active or less attentive than others only in certain situations, as for example in a classroom with its social distractions, or conversely at a time when cognitive or attentional demands are being made. *Shaffer et al.* (1974) examined this possibility by comparing neurologically normal and abnormal groups with and without a conduct disorder in two different settings. In one, children were invited to play with a number of different toys ranged out over a testing room, and motor activity and attention shifts were recorded. In the other the children performed a vigilance task and were instructed to sit still (on a chair which recorded wriggling movements). It was found that neurological state did not influence attention or activity in either situation. The children with a conduct disorder, regardless of associated neurological disease, were more active and less attentive in both situations. In other words, inattention and overactivity appeared as nonspecific correlates of a conduct disorder rather than as a specific indicator of brain damage.

In summary, the *hyperactivity syndrome,* although described in the literature with seeming clarity and little ambiguity, is in reality a difficult clinical diagnosis to make in a reliable way. In an experimental situation where such problems can be overcome there is little evidence to support a specific association between its clinical features and neurological dysfunction.

Given these difficulties follow-up studies should be especially helpful in deciding whether the syndrome is a distinct clinical entity.

The Montreal group (*Minde et al.*, 1971, 1972; *Weiss et al.*, 1971, 1975) have published a series of follow-up studies on 2 cohorts of non-psychotic children of normal intelligence, who had been reported to be overactive, both at home and at school, when originally referred for treatment between the ages of 6 and 13. The group as a whole had a high prevalence of early perinatal difficulties and scored poorly on the Lincoln Oseretsky scale of motor attainments. Over 90% of the subjects were boys and mean IQ was 103. There was minimal attrition from the original sample and outcome evaluation has included time-sampled classroom behaviour observations for a sub-group and standardised parent and teacher questionnaires and interviews used for evaluations both at the start of the study and at follow-up.

When seen in their teens, these boys were rated as being considerably less overactive than they had been in middle childhood. However, direct observation showed that they remained more active and distractible than same aged controls. Their patterns of *activity* had also altered. Whereas previously they had shown a deal of gross motor activity – hopping up and down from their school desks, walking around the classroom, etc. – they now differed primarily in being more fidgety. Boys who had earlier been very aggressive, were now less so, but one quarter of the sample were now judged to be antisocial. At psychiatric interview the dominant affect was sadness, an awareness of failure and low expectations for the future. These feelings were clearly well founded for 80% of the group had failed in class at least once and they were doing poorly on most subjects. This remained true even when the hyperactives were closely paired with controls on the same IQ. Mean motor performance on the Lincoln Oseretsky had declined since first testing but this did not seem to be reflected in everyday activities. On the whole the *hyperactives* did well at sport and in handicrafts.

The workers looked at predictive variables within the groups and good outcome was related to high IQ, the development of sociopathic traits to the earlier presence of family problems. Although they claim that neurological status at the outset did not influence final outcome, it is not clear from the published reports whether this is after taking account of IQ and family pathology, etc. Results are not expressed separately for children with and without soft signs or abnormal anamnesis.

The Montreal studies used a standardised initial assessment with which direct comparison was later possible. Other studies which have looked at Natural History have located their samples by a search of case records. Information in case records is of course rarely uniform, either in scope or calibration, and this makes these studies of less value. *Mendelson et al.* (1971) followed up 83 12- to 16-year-old adolescents whose notes revealed the presence of *hyperactivity* between 2 and 5 years previously. The study is uncontrolled, the original sample included children with an IQ ranging from 60 to 120 and many of the children came from broken homes or had sociopathic parents. No information is provided about neurological status. At follow-up a high proportion of the adolescents were moody, lacked confidence, had failed at school or had been in trouble with the police. Studies of this sort are of only limited value in our search for confirmation of a distinct minimal brain damage syndrome, for their initial constitution is almost certainly heterogenous and it is not possible to dissect out any necessary components which might affect outcome.

There have been two studies which have looked at the outcome in adult life. In both studies the diagnosis of hyperactivity was made retrospectively from routine clinical notes. *Menkes et al.* (1967) studied 14 cases who had earlier attended a paediatric neurology clinic. The average age at follow-up was 24 years. All had been described as *hyperactive* and had experienced *learning difficulties.* A variable number had been clumsy or had language difficulties, 4 had an IQ of less than 80 and a further 3 an IQ of between 80 and 90. 13 came from disturbed families. At follow-up – which was uncontrolled – the group had done poorly. Only half were self-supporting, 4 were institutionalised and psychotic and 2 were retarded.

Borland and Heckman (1976) has carried out a controlled study in which comparison was made between 20 men of average IQ who had been seen earlier at a child guidance clinic, where they had been described as overactive and inattentive, and their unaffected male siblings. Most came from good and stable families. Their mean age at re-examination was 30. The probands did not differ from their brothers in either work or marital adjustment and all were self-supporting. However, 4 probands, but no sibs were regarded as sociopathic using *Robins*'s (1966) criteria. The probands described themselves as being more restless and more frequently said that they had difficulty in sitting through a TV programme. They had experienced more job changes which they attributed to discontent with previous employment and a drive for self-improvement. A more detailed analysis of their work record showed that whilst at age 20 they had occupied jobs significantly lower in status than their brothers at the same age, the gap had narrowed during the 3rd decade. 50% of the male offspring of the probands had behaviour problems or difficulties at school compared to only 16% of the male offspring of the unaffected sibs.

It seems likely that the very different outcome reflected in these two follow-up studies among adults is a consequence of sample selection, thus highlighting some of the methodological difficulties referred to above.

Conclusions

Regretfully the contribution of these various follow-up studies to our knowledge of either a hypothetical MBD or hyperactivity syndrome is limited.

There is no evidence that children with a history of early perinatal complications but who have no evidence of persistent, conventionally elicited neurological abnormalities are predisposed to later social or psychological difficulties. However, definitive studies using early indices of neurological states and controlling for later environmental influences have yet to be done. The fact that behaviour disturbance appears to be increased in children with a history of head injury but with no apparent neurological abnormality would support the notion that undetectable brain damage may nevertheless influence learning ability or behaviour.

The inclusion criteria in even the best of the studies on so-called 'hyperactives' take little account of the inherent unreliability of parents or teachers judgements of overactivity. The samples are heterogenous and include children with a wide range of IQs, and degree of disturbance at home, and include children with and without organic indicators such as an abnormal anamnesis or the presence of soft signs. Although there is some consistency in the way that these studies indicate moderate social difficulties in later life, we cannot tell whether these are non-specific findings common to many children who experience early school failure or whether they are the consequence of more specific biological influences on behavioural style or mood.

In many ways it has been the studies of adult psychiatric disorder in patients with neurological soft signs, which have provided the most weighty support for the syndrome of MBD. The assumption being, of course, that the signs have persisted since childhood. If so, these subjects are presenting with seemingly distinctive forms of psychiatric illness in adolescence and adult life and are thus fulfilling one of the requirements of a clinically useful syndrome, i.e., that it should enable predictions to be made about outcome. However, further support is required, as for example by investigations into the prevalence of soft signs and psychiatric disturbance in an unselected adult or adolescent population, follow-up studies which differentiate between children with and without soft signs and by longitudinal research into children with soft signs to identify both the frequency with which one can expect signs to disappear (and ? appear *de novo*) and to note whether individuals with enduring or novel signs differ also in other respects.

Follow-up investigations have both clinical and theoretical value and hopefully adequately documented research in this area will continue and will eventually help us to define useful and meaningful diagnostic groups.

Summary

The concept of minimal brain damage has been the subject of a good deal of justified criticism. One method of validating the syndrome might to be undertake studies of the natural history of children in whom the diagnosis had been made to investigate whether outcome could be predicted from the presence or absence of one or more of its components. No studies exist to allow an exercise of this sort. The literature has, therefore been reviewed to examine the long-term social and behavioural sequelae of mild perinatal hazard, transient disturbances of CNS function, non-localizing ('soft') CNS signs and the hyperactivity syndrome.

It is concluded that apparently transient disturbances of the CNS may be followed by adverse behavioural sequelae which persist in the absence of other 'hard' neurological features and, further, that there is accumulating but, as yet incomplete, evidence that the presence of certain 'soft' neurological signs may determine the form of any later psychiatric disturbance.

References

Adams, R.M.; Kocsis, J.J., and Estes, R.E.: Soft neurological signs in learning-disabled children and controls. Am. J. Dis. Child. *128:* 614–618 (1974).

Black, P.; Jeffries, J.J.; Blumer, D.; Wellner, A., and Walker, A.: The post-traumatic syndrome in children; in *Walker, Caveness and Critchley* The late effects of head injury (Thomas, Springfield 1969).

Borland, B.L. and Heckman, H.K.: Hyperactive boys and their brothers. Archs gen. Psychiat. *33:* 669–675 (1976).

Burde, B. de la and Choate, M.S.: Does asymptomatic lead exposure in children have latent sequelae? J. Pediat. *81:* 1088–1091 (1972).

Burde, B. de la and Choate, M.S.: Early asymptomatic lead exposure and development at school age. J. Pediat. *87:* 638–642 (1975).

Butler, N.R. and Alberman, E.D.: Perinatal problems (Livingstone, Edinburgh 1969).

Chamberlain, R.; Chamberlain, C.; Howlett, B., and Claireaux, A.: British births 1970, vol. 1. The first week of life (Heinemann, London 1976).

Clements, S.D. and Peters, J.E.: Minimal brain dysfunction in the school age child. Archs gen. Psychiat. *6:* 185–197 (1962).

Craft, A.W.; Shaw, D.A., and Cartlidge, N.E.: Head injuries in children. Br. med. J. *iii:* 200–203 (1972).

Cravioto, J. and Delicardie, E.R.: Environmental correlates of severe clinical malnutrition and language development in survivors from Kwashiorkor or marasmus. Nutrition, the nervous system and behaviour. Proc. Semin. Malnutrition in Early Life and Subsequent Mental Development, Mona 1972.

Davie, R.; Butler, N., and Goldstein, H.: From birth to seven. A report of the national child developmental study (Longman, London 1972).

Dodge, P.R. and Swartz, M.N.: Bacterial meningitis; a review of selected aspects. II. Special neurological problems, post-meningitis complications and clinicopathological correlations. New Engl. J. Med. *272:* 954–960 (1965).

Ellis, C.E. and Hill, D.E.: Growth, intelligence and school performance in children with cystic fibrosis who have had an episode of malnutrition during infancy. J. Pediat. *87:* 565–568 (1975).

Fisch, R.O.; Bilek, M.S.; Horrobin, J.M., and Chang, P.: Children with superior intelligence at 7 years of age. Am. J. Dis. Child. *130:* 481–487 (1976).

Gibbs, F.; Gibbs, E.; Spies, H., and Carpenter, P.: Common types of childhood encephalitis. Archs Neurol. *10:* 1–11 (1964).

Gottfried, A.W.: Intellectual consequences of perinatal anoxia. Psychol. Bull. *80:* 231–242 (1973).

Graham, F.K.; Ernhard, C.B.; Thurston, C.B., and Craft, M.: Development three years after perinatal anoxia and other potentially damaging newborn experiences. Psychol. Monogr. *76:* 1–53 (1962).

Hertzig, M.A. and Birch, H.G.: Neurologic organisation in psychiatrically disturbed adolescent girls. Archs gen. Psychiat. *15:* 590–599 (1966).

Hjern, B. and Nylander, I.: Acute head injuries in children. Traumatology, therapy and prognosis. Acta paediat. scand., suppl. 152 (1964).

Kalverboer, A.F.; Touwen, B.C., and Prechtl, H.F.: Follow-up of infants at risk of minor brain dysfunction. Ann. N.Y. Acad. Sci. *205:* 173–187 (1973).

Kennard, M.: Value of equivocal signs in neurological diagnosis. Neurology, Minneap. *10:* 753–764 (1960).

Klein, P.S.S.; Forbes, G.B., and Nader, P.R.: Effects of starvation in infancy (pyloric stenosis) on subsequent learning abilities. J. Pediat. *87:* 8–15 (1975).

Klonoff, H. and Paris, R.: Immediate, short term and residual effects of acute head injuries in children. Neuropsychological and neurological correlates; in *Reiton and Davidson* Clinical neuropsychology. Current status and applications (Halstead Press, New York 1974).

Knobloch, H. and Pasamanick, B.: Prospective studies on the epidemiology of reproductive casualty. Methods, findings and some implications. Merrill-Palmer Q. behav. Dev. *12:* 27–43 (1966).

Lansdown, R.G.; Shepher, J.; Clayton, B.E.; Delves, H.T.; Graham, P.J., and Turner, W.S.: Blood levels. Behaviour and intelligence: a population study. Lancet *i:* 538–541 (1974).

Lapouse, R. and Monk, M.A.: An epidemiologic study of behavioural characteristics in children. Am. J. publ. Hlth *48:* 1134–1144 (1958).

Mannheimer, D.I. and Mellinger, G.D.: Personality characteristics of the child accident repeater. Child Dev. *38:* 491–513 (1967).

Mendelson, W.; Johnson, N., and Stewart, M.: Hyperactive children as teen-agers. A follow-up study. J. nerv. ment. Dis. *153:* 273–279 (1971).

Menkes, M.; Rowe, J., and Menkes, J.: A 25-year follow-up study on the hyperkinetic child with minimal brain dysfunction. Pediatrics, Springfield *39:* 393–399 (1967).

Minde, K.; Lewin, D.; Weiss, G., et al.: Studies on the hyperactive child. VIII. 5-year follow-up. Archs gen. Psychiat. *24:* 409–414 (1971).

Minde, K.; Weiss, G., and Mendelson, N.: A 5 year follow-up study of 91 hyperactive school children. J. Am. Acad. Child Psychiat. *11:* 595–610 (1972).

Mosher, L.R.; Pollin, W., and Stabenau, J.R.: Identical twins discordant for schizophrenia. Archs gen. Psychiat. *24:* 422–430 (1971).

Muller, R.; Nylander, I., and Larrson, L.E.: Sequelae of primary aseptic meningo-encephalitis. A clinical sociomedical electroencephalographic and psychological study. Acta psychiat. scand., suppl. 126, pp. 1–115 (1958).

Myklebust, H.R.: Identification and diagnosis of children with learning disabilities. An interdisciplinary study of criteria. Semin. Psychiat. *5:* 55–77 (1973).

Peters, J.E.; Roming, J.S., and Dykman, R.A.: A special neurological examination of children with learning disabilities. Devl Med. Child Neurol. *175:* 63–75 (1975).

Prechtl, H.F.: Prognostic value of neurological signs in the newborn infant. Proc. R. Soc. Med. *58:* 3–4 (1965).

Quitkin, F.; Rifkin, A., and Klein, D.F.: Neurologic soft signs in schizophrenia and character disorder. Archs gen. Psychiat. *33:* 845–853 (1976).

Robins, L.N.: Deviant children grown up (Williams & Wilkins, Baltimore 1966).

Rochford, J.M.; Detre, T.; Tucker, G.J., and Harrow, M.: Neuropsychological impairments in functional psychiatric disease. Archs gen. Psychiat. *22:* 114–119 (1970).

Rutter, M.; Graham, P., and Birch, H.G.: Interrelations between choreiform syndrome, reading disability and psychiatric disorder in children of 8–11 years. Devl Med. Child Neurol. *8:* 149–159 (1966).

Rutter, M.; Graham, P., and Yule, W.: A neuropsychiatric study in childhood. Clins in dev. Med., No. 35/36 (SIMP/Heinemann, London 1970a).

Rutter, M.; Tizard, J., and Whitmore, K.: Education, health and behaviour (Longman, London 1970b).

Sells, C.J.; Carpenter, R.L., and Ray, C.G.: Sequelae of central nervous system enterovirus infections. New Engl. J. Med. *293:* 1–4 (1975).

Schulman, J.L.; Kaspar, J.C., and Throne, F.M.: Brain damage and behaviour. A clinical-experimental study (Thomas, Springfield 1965).

Shaffer, D.; McNamara, N., and Pincus, J.: Controlled observations on patterns of activity, attention and impulsivity in brain damaged and psychiatrically disturbed boys. Psychol. Med. *4:* 4–18 (1974).

Shaffer, D.; Chadwick, O., and Rutter, M.: Psychiatric outcome of localised head injury in children; in *Porter and Fitzsimons* Outcome of severe damage to the central nervous system. CIBA Foundation Symposium No. 34 (Elsevier-Excerpta Medica-North Holland, Amsterdam 1975).

Stine, O.C.; Saratsiotis, J.M., and Mosser, R.S.: Relationships between neurological findings and classroom behaviour. Am. J. Dis. Child. *129:* 1036–1040 (1975).

Strauss, A.A. and Lehtinen, L.E.: Psychopathology and education of the brain injured child, vol. 1 (Grune & Stratton, New York 1947).

Ucko, L.E.: A comparative study of asphyxiated and nonasphyxiated boys from birth to 5 years. Devl Med. Child Neurol. *7:* 643–657 (1965).

Weiss, G.; Minde, K.; Werry, J.S., et al.: Studies of the hyperactive child. Archs gen. Psychiat. *24:* 409–414 (1971).

Weiss, G.; Kruger, E.; Danielson, U., and Elman, M.: Effect of long term treatment of hyperactive children with methylphenidate. Can. med. Ass. J. *112:* 159–165 (1975).

Wender, P.: The minimal brain dysfunction syndrome in children. J. nerv. ment. Dis. *155:* 55–71 (1972).

Werner, E.; Bierman, J.M.; French, F.E., et al.: Reproductive and environmental casualties. A report on the 10-year follow-up of the children of the Kuai pregnancy study. Pediatrics, Springfield *42:* 112–127 (1968).

Werry, J.S.; Minde, K.; Guzman, A.; Weiss, G.; Dogan, K., and Hoy, E.: Neurological status compared with neurotic and normal children. Am. J. Orthopsychiat. *42:* 441–451 (1972).

Wolff, P.H. and Hurwitz, J.: The choreiform syndrome. Devl Med. Child Neurol. *8:* 160–165 (1966).

Wolff, p.H. and Hurwitz, J.: Functional implications of the mentally brain damaged syndrome. Semin. Psychiat. *5:* 105–115 (1973).

D. Shaffer, MB, MRCP, MRC Psych., Director, Division of Child Psychiatry, Department of Psychiatry, New York Psychiatric Institute, 722 West 168th Street, *New York, NY 10032* (USA)

Adv. biol. Psychiat., vol. 1, pp. 35–54 (Karger, Basel 1978)

Diagnosis: Developmental Psychological Assessment

William Yule
University of London Institute of Psychiatry, London

Introduction

A few years ago, *Conners* (1973) said that 'In surveying this literature on the clinical utility of psychological tests, it is remarkable how uniform is the opinion of the reviewers that it is both logically and empirically unwarranted for psychological tests to serve as practical tools in making individual diagnostic decisions about underlying brain pathology in children.' Yet, nearly 5 years later, I have been asked to talk to the title 'Diagnosis: Developmental Psychological Assessment', and there have been countless studies published in the interim where psychological tests have been used in the study of children with so-called 'Minimal Brain Dysfunction'. How can *Conners'* conclusion be reconciled with current practice, and how can current practice be improved?

It is the aim of this paper to clarify some of the confusions which surround the practice of diagnosing MBD in children. I will argue that the concept of MBD is now so overinclusive as to be more harmful than helpful in clinical practice. Nevertheless, there are many children whose very real learning and behavioural difficulties will not disappear just because they get reclassified by a different label. Therefore, I will argue, the role of psychological assessment in this area is to provide much more detailed and precise descriptions of current levels of functioning. From a clinical point of view, such information should ultimately carry implications for therapeutic intervention. At a theoretical level, such detailed data should permit the identification of more discrete, better defined sub-groups from among the heterogeneous population labelled MBD.

Since the aims of the clinician who wants to help the individual child are different from the aims of the researcher who is interested in furthering our understanding of brain behaviour relationships, it is little wonder that attempts to apply findings from one area to problems in another have resulted in much confusion. Ultimately, clinicians have to apply research findings to single cases, but hitherto this has been done almost intuitively, as an art form. Recently, there has been a resurgence of interest in experimental methods which can be applied rigorously to the study of single cases (*Yule and Hemsley,* 1977) and this paper will conclude by arguing that the application of such methods to the investigation and treatment of individual children presenting with learning and behavioural difficulties will illuminate both clinical-therapeutic and theoretical issues.

The Concept of 'Minimal Brain Dysfunction'

Before one can discuss diagnosis, one has to be clear about the condition one is attempting to diagnose. It seems to me that some of the confusions surrounding MBD can be understood in terms of the history of the development of the concept.

For many years, parents and teachers have been concerned about children who were 'not doing as well as expected', who were overactive, or who were just a little bit different from normal. The fashion among professionals in the 1930s dictated that such difficulties be interpreted along psychoanalytic lines. This may have resulted in many creative interpretations, but it did little to help solve the children's problems. Then, with the remarkable developments in adult neuropsychology which demonstrated the behavioural sequelae of various discrete brain injuries, the brain was again considered as being responsible for many of the difficulties presented by the children. Neurologists, psychologists and teachers all incorporated this notion into their separate conceptual systems, and the result has been the concept of 'minimal brain dysfunction'. Let us examine some of the fallacies that underly the development of this concept as I have outlined it:

(1) Since children are developing organisms, it is erroneous to apply the findings of studies of adults with mature brains to the study of children. As *Conners* (1973) puts it: '... it seems reasonable to assume that subtle deviations of the nervous system in young and developing organisms will present more complex relationships at a behavioral level than with older individuals or subjects who have sustained clearly defined cerebral insults.'

(2) Most neuropsychological studies of adults proceed from the knowledge of brain damage in the patient to identifying and analysing the behavioural consequences of that known damage (*Benton,* 1973). It is fallacious to argue that because injury in brain-site A is followed by behavioural deficit B, then that identification of deficit B implies injury A.

(3) With children, it has become common to imply 'dysfunction' in a particular area rather than 'damage'. This does nothing to get away from the dilemma that here, the neuropsychologist is involved in the revere process from that with adults. He has to infer damage or dysfunction at a cerebral level from a study of the child's observable behaviour. Thus, as *Benton* (1973) puts it,

' "Minimal brain dysfunction" is a behavioral concept with neurological implications'.

Partly as a result of faulty reasoning as described above, it became common practice in some quarters to diagnose 'brain damage' on the basis of psychological test patterns found previously in adult patients, or on the basis of uncertain neurological evidence (so-called 'soft signs') or on the basis of the presence of overactivity and other behaviours. The net result has been voluminous writings on 'the MBD child'.

The most common characteristics of MBD have been listed as: '... hyperactivity (hyperkinesis); perceptual-motor impairments; emotional lability; general co-ordination defects; disorders of attention (e.g. short attention span, distractibility, perseveration); disorders of impulse and inhibition; disorders of thinking (ideation) and memory; specific learning disabilities, e.g., reading, dyslexias, arithmetic, spelling; disorders of speech and hearing; equivocal neurological signs and electro-encephalographic (EEG) irregularities' (*Becker,* 1976) – *Ingram* (1973) also reprints the same list, but he acknowledges that it was issued by a drug company.

Becker (1976) quite unintentionally illustrates what is wrong with regarding MBD as a diagnostic syndrome of any value. He tries to give a clinical description of how the child with MBD may initially present to the clinician. The child may be '... clumsy, awkward, anxious, fidgety, angry or restless ... excessively physically active ... temper tantrums ... sensitive ...' and so on. After listing many more than 50 adjectives which are a muddle of description and interpretation, *Becker* makes the classic admission, 'Interestingly, some children with MBD may be behaviourally quite different'! There then follows a list of the opposite adjectives.

It is loose, overinclusive thinking such as this which made *Ingram* (1973) conclude that ' "Minimal brain damage" is not a diagnosis; it is an escape from making one ... the use of the terms "soft signs" and "minimal brain damage" is diagnostic of soft thinking. These terms should be discarded. Paediatricians should describe what they find. Then they should evaluate their findings and state the inferences they draw from their evaluation of their findings.'

In other words, MBD is the great egalitarian disorder – anyone and everyone has it. Even if conservative estimates are used and it is considered that 15–20% of a group of children have MBD, I would argue that it is more dangerous in our present knowledge to regard such a large group as having dysfunctions in common that it is to treat each child individually. Over inclusive diagnostic categories conceal more individual variation than they reveal. Children develop the sort of problems alluded to above for many reasons. Thus, the MBD syndrome is dangerous because (a) it implies a homogeneous symptomatology, and (b) it implies a known aetiology, namely some form of brain damage or dysfunction. It is clear that the current evidence does not support either of these propositions.

This is the position adopted by *Benton* (1973) who then argues that what is needed is for the heterogeneous groups to be studied in greater detail so that new sub-groupings can be identified. *Cohen* (1973, 1976) goes further, he claims, not unreasonably as we have seen, that the MBD label is useless. He points out that all that the clinician or the researcher can do is observe and code the child's behaviour. 'Brain dysfunction', 'intelligence', 'attention', 'hyperkinesis' and so on are all abstract concepts. They do not exist. They are inferred from detailed observations. Thus, from a different standpoint *Cohen* agrees with *Ingram* and to some extent with *Benton* that in studying children with supposed MBD we need really to study their behaviour in much more specific detail.

This argument and approach is not as nihilistic as some neuropsychologists may fear at first hearing it. None of these writers, and certainly not the present author, is denying the existence of children with a wide variety of problems which appear to have a developmental/neurological component. Clumsy children do exist, so do bright children who have difficulty with reading or spelling. Overactive children exist, although maybe only in certain situations. We all recognize that children can display the behaviours alluded to by *Becker*. The point at issue is whether our understanding of these children's difficulties is helped by calling them MBD. It is argued that there is a need to dispense with premature 'neurologizing', and to return to a situation where the problems presented by the child are adequately *described* before they are interpreted. Such descriptions need to be in precise, behavioural terms. 'Signs', 'symptoms', 'delays' – all of them need to be operationally defined and there is a need to find means of measuring them objectively and reliably.

Thus, what is good advice for Dr. *Ingram*'s paediatrician is also good advice for the psychologist who intends helping children with real if ill-understood developmental and neurological and behavioural difficulties.

What is Meant by 'Diagnosis'

In this spirit of critically examining concepts and trying to operationalize them, let us examine what is meant by 'making a diagnosis'. Immediately, a source of confusion is identified since different professional groups can use the term in distinct ways – the neurologist may wish information to assist in identifying or excluding the presence of a recognizable brain disorder; the teacher may wish to know what are the child's cognitive strengths and weaknesses, and what limitations, if any, are placed on future progress by the child's (inferred) medical condition. Little wonder that working in multi-professional groups in children's clinics is so difficult – different professionals require data for different purposes. Alas, all too often they try to be nice to each other and use each others terms, but in their own ways!

Thus, a diagnosis is made with a purpose – even if that purpose is not always made explicit. Someone notices that the child is having difficulty either at home or at school. The child is referred for expert diagnosis. The expectation of the referral agents is that the experts will tell them what is wrong with the child and what to do about it. Thus, information is needed to satisfy a number of questions, but the primary need is for a much more precise description of the presenting problem. Most clinicians are tempted to make inferences about causation, but all too often information is not gathered with the clear purpose of providing guidance on how best to help the child.

Notice, however, that this approach to diagnosis is problem oriented. The sort of investigations undertaken, the sort of assessments that are carried out will, to a very large extent, be determined by the problem as originally presented and by the information needed to help formulate treatment goals. That is not to say that the clinician ignores other problems presented by the child, of course not. He will make brief enquiries during history taking of many aspects relating to the child's overall development. But it means that the focus of investigation must remain the presenting problem.

This approach, from the psychologist's point of view, is very much individual centred and is therefore at odds with the battery-testing approach used by such North American and Canadian investigators as *Reitan and Heineman* (1968), *Doehring* (1968) and *Rourke* (1975, 1976). In fairness, these investigators are interested in conducting research into brain behaviour relationships rather than investigating children from a clinically service point of view. However, it is advisable to note the different aims of the two approaches, since, at times, psychologists in clinics are under pressure to use such broad batteries with every case.

Developmental Psychological Assessment

At present, developmental psychological assessment is in a peculiar state. Assessments consist of a mixture of standardized tests – some with sound theoretical bases, others with no theoretical basis – and quasi-experimental techniques. Criterion referenced tasks exist alongside standardized instruments, and no two groups of workers agree on which form of assessment is most useful for what purpose. Too often assessment is seen as an end in itself, and little thought is given to providing evidence which has implications for treatment. It is difficult to discuss these issues without reference to particular clinical problems. Nevertheless, I will try to clarify broad principles before focusing on specific procedures.

The Need for Standardized Tests

It is very old-fashioned these days to talk of tests, their standardization, reliability and validity. Nonetheless, such tools still have an important, if circumscribed role in assessing children. Since the children we are discussing today frequently present with developmental difficulties, it is important to know how they compare on particular functions with children of the same age. Standardized tests allow one to say not only whether a child is performing less well than his age-peers, but also they provide *quantitative* information regarding the extent of the deficit.

Whether or not a child who scores 1 SD below the mean on the Oseretsky Test of Motor Proficiency should be categorized as a 'clumsy' child becomes an empirical matter. Test scores derive their validity solely from empirical studies. But at least the existence of a few standardized tests of important developmental functions greatly reduces the subjective element in clinical examinations.

Criterion Referenced Tests

However, standardized tests which yield age norms are often very crude instruments – crude in the sense that they measure many functions simultaneously and the end score is the result of the operation of many psychological processes. At times, one needs to know more simply whether a particular behaviour exists or not in the child's repertoire.

Such all-or-none 'tests' correspond roughly to the more classical paediatric-neurological examination. Since this has been well described and developed by the authors, I will not touch on it more at this stage (*Touwen and Prechtl,* 1970; *Rutter, et al.*, 1970a; *Kalverboer,* 1975).

To illustrate criterion referenced testing in other areas, let us look briefly at reading and language development:

Reading. Usually, when considering the problems children present in reading, psychologists first administer a standardized test which, if well selected, will provide information on both the child's accuracy of reading and his comprehension of reading. However, the remedial teacher may be more interested in the child's phonic 'word-attack' skills. Can the child produce the commonest sound value when he sees a particular letter? Does he name each letter appropriately? Does he know a particular rule of pronunciation?

It would be possible to list a whole range of small, discrete skills, all of which go to producing the higher-order skill we call reading. In effect, this is what teachers try to do – the inefficiency lying in the fact that most teachers do so in their own way and so cannot compare findings.

Language. The revolution in our understanding of children's language development since developmental psycholinguistics appeared in the last decade, has meant that even language skills can be broken down into small, discrete steps. I have argued elsewhere that this information can be utilized in planning remedial programmes (*Yule and Berger,* 1975), but it should be emphasized here that it can also be used to pinpoint which skills a child has in his repertoire.

For example, *Palermo* (1970) notes that there is a close relationship between the morpheme-length-of-utterance and the appearance of rules of negatives and interrogatives. This observation can be used in pinpointing language disorders by firstly noting the length of the child's utterance and then checking to see whether the structures one would expect to find normally are present in his repertoire. This, of course, is an illustration of how a normative, standardized approach can be complementary to our ipsative, criterion referenced approach.

These two brief examples also make another point clear. That is that criterion referenced testing yields information which is much more relevant therapeutically. Once the assessor has listed those skills which a child has attained, he has provided a detailed description of the child's behaviour. But he has done much more. He has provided a baseline against which future progress (or deterioration) can be measured, and where the skills are hierarchical in nature such as in language and reading (*Staats,* 1968) he has indicated the goals of future treatment.

The Theoretical Basis of Tests

Although pragmatists might argue that the theoretical basis on which a test is constructed is irrelevant to its later use, provided the relevant empirical data are available, it is as well to see the effects of the test constructors' theoretical model on the diagnostic value of the data. Again, let us take an example from the area of language.

One of the best-known, not to say notorious, tests of language is the Illinois Test of Psycholinguistic Ability (*Kirk et al.,* 1968). This was deliberately constructed to assess the different components of *Osgood*'s (1957) now outmoded model of language. Independent empirical studies using factor analytic techniques (*Mittler and Ward,* 1970) have shown that there is indeed one general factor which can be identified as 'language', but the other subtests do not appear to be tapping discrete functions. Thus, a complicated test yields a single, global, usable measure according to the empirical studies. Yet the literature is full of unsophisticated studies which gleefully interpret ITPA profiles and base remedial programmes on nothing more substantial than random error variance.

Another ill-fated – or rather, psychometrically inadequate – test is the Frostig Developmental Test of Visual Perception (*Frostig et al.,* 1964). Again it claims to assess five separate aspects of visuo-motor skills, and a whole industry has built up around this test. The test profile guides the remedial programme, and both are scarcely worth the paper they are printed on. The test itself does not stand up to psychometric investigation, in that factorial studies fail to confirm the independence of the subscales, and in any case the scale is highly related to general intelligence (*Berger and Yule,* 1972; *Olson,* 1968). Furthermore, the evidence shows that training of perceptual skills by the Frostig-Horne method merely increases the scores on the Frostig test. There is no carry over to reading skills.

These two salutory tales are presented as instances where tests were developed to fit a particular model, but were not abandoned when evidence demonstrated that they were not doing what they were meant to do. Moreover, it should be noted that the existence of the tests and the underlying theoretical assumption (in the case of the Frostig test) that visuo-perceptual deficits underlay reading problems, may actually have prevented children from getting appropriate remedial help. If you want to teach a child to read, teach him a subskill of reading – not how to balance on beams, trace along curved lines or whatever (*Yule,* 1976; *Cohen,* 1976).

In fairness, it might be said that the above examples illustrate the lack of training and sophistication of the professionals who misuse readymade assessment tools rather than think for themselves. Nevertheless, the danger of wrongly using tests of any sort must be recognised.

General Intelligence

Nowhere was this cautionary note more needed than in the field of testing general intelligence. Despite the fact that its weaknesses (*Berger,* 1970) have led to its being abandoned in our own Institute, the Standford Binet is still widely used. Many people appear still to be unaware of its strong verbal bias. It is still not uncommon to see children with specific language disorders being classified as generally mentally retarded because their general intelligence was wrongly assessed on a highly verbal test such as the Binet.

I believe that it is still very valuable to get an estimate of the child's general level of intelligence – but both his verbal and non-verbal IQ on a test such as the *WISC.* This is because a well-standardised test of general intelligence gives a relatively unbiased estimate of the child's current level of functioning over a wide range of skills which are not directly taught. Too often, parents' and teachers' expectations are based on their observation of an isolated skill or an isolated deficit which appears under particular conditions. An external assessment can sometimes clarify the situation.

Notice that I am *not* saying that the parents or teachers were incorrect in their observations. What I am saying is that their observations may be incomplete, in a large part because children's behaviour is so situation specific. A test of general intelligence is, of course, not free from social and cultural influence, but compared to the observations of most teachers, it is *relatively* free from situational effects. Hence its value as part of a comprehensive assessment procedure. Where there are discrepancies between the results obtained in a psychological assessment and those reported by the teachers or parents, such discrepancies should be further investigated, not dismissed or ignored.

I will return later to the use of profile indices obtained from intelligence tests. Here, I would like to point to one other pervasive problem. As noted earlier, tests like the WISC have little theoretical basis. They were developed as the result of accumulated wisdom, mythology and prejudice over many years. Like any information, the test scores on WISC subtests are open to many interpretations. Factor analytic studies have broadly confirmed the existence of a general factor, a verbal factor and a visuo-spatial factor. Unfortunately, many psychologists have attempted to infer things from the WISC subscales that are not really warranted. For example, it is frequently claimed that scores on the Digit Span and Arithmetic subscales reflect 'attention span' (*Bortner,* 1968). Now, it may well be that some factorial studies show these two subtests to relate together and it may be that compared to the other subscales an armchair content analysis suggests that what they have in common is something to do with attention and concentration, but this does not mean that the two scales are good or even useful measures of such behaviour. In fact, other studies suggest that scores on the two subscales relate very poorly to other measures of attention (*Kassinove and Summers,* 1968).

The way I suggest such composite scales be used is as follows: The psychologist must be aware of the literature which has attempted to analyse the content of the subscales (*Sattler,* 1974). He needs to know about the unreliability of such short scales and also how to assess whether a difference between two scores is reliable and abnormal (*Payne and Jones,* 1957). Together, these sorts of information will help him formulate hypotheses to account for his observations. The hypotheses need to be tested further on other tests or experimental procedures.

Thus, I am arguing that I believe that tests of general intelligence still have an important role in assessing children referred because of developmental or behavioural problems. They allow the psychologist to obtain a relatively unbiased estimate of the child's overall development which is then interpreted against information from other sources. Agreements and discrepancies in this information allow more specific hypotheses to be formulated and appropriate further investigation can then be undertaken.

Situation-Specificity

As more and more psychologists have returned to observing children's behaviour in its natural setting, so they have re-discovered one of the fundamental problems of human psychology. In undergraduate courses, the problem is usually referred to as one of 'generalisability' in an experimental setting. Students are cautioned that they can only generalise results to other groups to the extent that the groups belong to the same parent population. As most critical studies of the MBD literature have noted, samples of children studied are rarely drawn appropriately from a parent population. Epidemiological studies are few and far between.

This aspect of 'generalisation' is by now reasonably well documented. However, another aspect of the same problem is less well recognised. Behaviour that is seen under testing conditions in the clinic may not be typical of the child's behaviour in other, more natural settings. Thus, one may not be able to generalise findings from the clinic to the real-life setting.

Evidence for this statement comes from a number of sources. From the field of behaviour modification, it has been noted that new skills learned in the laboratory do not automatically transfer to other settings. Generalisation has to be worked for (*Patterson and Brodsky,* 1966). In our own epidemiological studies, we found that parents and teachers could each yield reliable ratings of children's behaviour. However, the two groups identified different children or showing disturbance at home or at school (*Rutter et al.,* 1970).

More central to the present symposium, 'hyperactivity' has been found to be highly situation-specific. Leaving aside for the moment the problem of formulating an objective measure of 'hyperactivity', careful studies have shown that most children who are reported to be overactive at school show no evidence of overactivity at home or in the clinic. For example, *Klein and Gittelman-Klein* (1975) studied 155 children reported to be overactive in school. Only 25% of these were found to be overactive in the home and the clinic settings as well. Hyperactivity was rarely witnessed in the clinic. Like aggression (*Bandura,* 1973), hyperactivity is a construct which may tell more about the level of tolerance of the labeller than it does about the actual behaviour of the child who is so labelled.

Further evidence of situation-specificity comes from *Kalverboer*'s (1975) excellent observational study. It will be recalled that under the relatively minor environmental changes made within the same observational room, the children's behaviour altered not only dramatically, but also lawfully. This was a convincing demonstration that children's behaviour alters in response to relatively minor changes in their social and physical environment. Again, it argues for the need to be much more specific in setting up experiments, and much more cautious about generalising the results obtained from one setting to another. It is really not justifiable to generalise results from the artificial laboratory setting to the real-life classroom or home setting. At best, laboratory experimental findings serve as fruitful sources of hypothesis for experimental trials to be undertaken in the setting where the problem is manifested.

Some Important Developmental Measures

In this section, I would like to consider briefly some of the measures which have been proposed and used in the studies to date of MBD children.

Motor Behaviour

Usually, two broad categories of behaviour are considered under this heading – roughly corresponding to the concepts of 'clumsiness' and 'overactivity'.

Clearly these need to be considered separately, but less obviously, until it is pointed out, 'clumsiness' is also a hybrid concept. Take for example the various versions of the Oseretsky Test of Motor Proficiency (*Rutter et al.,* 1970a). It measures both gross and fine motor activity and yields overall scores which confound differences from different limbs and different sides of the body. Thus, while a test such as that is preferable to a teacher's or even a neurologists' rating of 'clumsiness', such a test can really only be regarded as a screening instrument.

Regarding overactivity, it has already been noted that this is a highly value laden construct. Even when attempts have been made to operationalise it, there is little agreement on which sort of hyperactivity to measure. *Sprague et al.* (1970) favoured sitting the child on a special seat where even minute movements could be recorded, whereas *Halverson and Waldrop* (1973) used a pedometer which failed to distinguish between MBD and normal children. As *Wender* (1975) notes, it may be that MBD children are not so much universally overactive, but rather that their level of activity is inappropriate to the situation they are in.

Attention

This is a concept which has proved elusive over many years. Whilst most previous writers regard attentional difficulties as being present in most, if not all MBD children, few define the construct. Sometimes they mean that the child has a short attention span, at other times they mean that he is highly distractable or that he cannot focus his attention on relevant stimuli for long. However, it is also noted (*Wender,* 1975) that in a one-to-one situation with plenty of positive reinforcement, such children show much fewer attention difficulties.

Ross (1976) has recently reviewed the literature on attention difficulties in children with learning difficulties. He argues very convincingly that more notice should be paid to measuring such childrens ability to show selective attention – the skill of limiting the number of stimuli that are processed at any one time. This is truly a developing ability and, most importantly for therapy, a skill which can be taught under appropriate conditions. For further discussions of attention in relation to learning disorders, see *Knights and Bakker* (1976).

Impulse Control

Although *Wender* (1975) describes poor impulse control as the most common referral complaint, it has always seemed strange to me that this should have been operationalised into the Matching Familiar Figures Test (*Kagan,* 1965). Whatever the processes measured in that test, and these are in doubt (*Block et al.,* 1974), the sort of impulsive response it measures is a far cry from the behaviour of the child who hits out in a rage and cannot control those sorts of impulses. Shared labels referring to different behaviours are, as always, confusing. Behavioural observational measures such as those proposed by *Patterson et al.* (1965) seem more relevant to the measurement of poor impulse control as usually understood.

Language

I have already commented on some of the difficulties of measuring language development with a test like the Illinois Test of Psycholinguistic Abilities. However, I think it is important that a number of different aspects of language development are assessed. More particularly, I believe that it is important to assess comprehension or understanding of language separately from the child's expressive use of language. Equally, I believe that assessment of the speech components – i.e. the mechanical, articulatory aspect – should be undertaken separately from the linguistic, cognitive components.

I have no very firm recommendations to make regarding the suitability of tests in these areas, partly because language tests travel badly across language barriers. However, in Britain we are finding the Reynell Developmental Language Scales (*Reynell,* 1969) which yield separate measures of comprehension and expressive language to be quite useful, although many more validation studies would be welcomed. The Edinburgh Articulation Test (*Anthony et al.,* 1971) is also a welcome addition to our testing armamentarium. The latter allows one to pin-point those irritating consonant substitutions which experienced testers can often notice, but not record.

Reading

Finally, I would like to say a word about the assessment of reading skills. An important point to remember is that the most relevant skills in reading change with age. Visual-motor-perceptual skills are relatively important in early stages; cognitive-linguistic skills are more important later. This is reflected in tests which place greater emphasis on the accuracy of reading at early stages, and correspondingly greater emphasis on comprehension later on. Remember, it is unusual to expect children over the age of 12 years or thereabouts to read out aloud, and many may make many errors of accuracy even though their understanding is unimpaired. In the middle years of schooling, tests which yield measures of both accuracy and comprehension are to be preferred to those which only call for the child to pronounce words out of context.

Some Recurring Psychometric Problems

In the space available, it is impossible to mention all the psychometric pitfalls that lie between testing and the interpretation of results. In this section, I will refer briefly to some of the major ones which occur in the messy area of assessing children with learning difficulties.

The Measurement of Underachievement

Most of the children we are concerned about in this conference are those who are 'not doing as well as is expected'. Apparently bright children are reading well below age level; good readers are making atrocious spelling errors; not very bright children seem unusually poor in language compared even to other dull children. In each case, one is making an implicit comparison of the same child on at least two different measures. Such comparisons are easily put into imprecise words; it is much more difficult to translate these simple concepts into quantifiable, operationalised measurements.

The major statistical pitfall which is embeded in the concept of this problem and its educational implications are admirably discussed in *Thorndike* (1963). Put simply, what is meant is as follows: No two tests of separate functions are perfectly correlated (they would not be separate functions if the correlation were unity!). Therefore, if a child scores high on one measure (say of general intelligence), while he may still score higher than the average on the second measure (say of reading), on average his score on the second measure will be less extreme than his score on the first. Thus, if you make a straight comparison between the measures and do not allow for this effect of regression to the mean, you are more likely to identify extremely intelligent children as underachievers. At the other end of the scale, you are more likely to identify extremely dull children as doing better than expected.

At present, the best way to avoid this problem is to use statistical techniques of regression analysis in selecting children who are doing less well than expected. My colleagues and I have used these procedures to good effect in our studies in the Isle of Wight and in London (*Yule,* 1967; *Rutter and Yule,* 1975; *Berger et al.,* 1975). The use of such techniques leads to the identification of much more specific subgroupings of children from among the population with heterogeneous learning disorders.

'Profile' Analysis

Ultimately, it may be one purpose of a psychometric assessment to pinpoint a child's strengths and weaknesses. However, it is necessary that each component measure should be both a reliable and a valid measure of the psychological process or skill in question. Where two tests are unreliable, differences between scores on the two tests will arise frequently as a result of errors of measurement. The shorter the test, the less reliable the resulting measure. Therefore, if two short tests are compared, it is highly likely that the same child will apparently score differently on each test. Let me give a concrete example.

The verbal and performance scales of the WISC are each reasonably reliable. Even so, differences of 9 points in either direction occur in over 50% of normal children aged $7^1/_2$ years. 10% of the population have differences as large as 22 points (*Field,* 1960). For a difference to be statistically abnormal, it has to be very large indeed, and mere statistical infrequency is no guarantee that the difference is clinically relevant (see below).

If this is the case with two lengthy scales such as the verbal and performance scales, how much more difficult it is to interpret differences between the much shorter (and hence much less reliable) individual subscales (*Hopkins,* 1964). Charting profiles on WISC, Frostig or ITPA is indeed a hazardous and misleading business (*Berger and Yule,* 1972).

WISC Verbal-Performance Discrepancies

While on the subject of 'profile' analysis, let me say a few words about the most widely used and abused diagnostic profile – the difference between scores on the WISC verbal and performance scales. I have discussed the development of this index more fully elsewhere (*Rutter et al.,* 1970a), and in many ways its history reflects the operation of all the fallacies discussed earlier.

The index developed from studies of adults with known brain damage. Groups of such subjects, when tested on the Wechsler-Bellevue, scored significantly higher *average* scores on the verbal than on the performance scale. Now the literature on how *groups* of children with heterogeneous, putative brain injury score on the WISC is confusing. Most studies compound many errors of biased case selection. However, the more important point to note here is that it is a big jump to argue that because a statistically significant difference of a few points occurs in groups of children, that in any individual child a small difference between the scales has any pathognomonic significance. What is needed are studies of large groups of children so that the distribution of differences can be examined. Even then, such information would be of limited value since the index is really needed when brain injury or dysfunction is suspected rather than known.

In our own study of brain-damaged children on the Isle of Wight, we produced some modest support for the view that a performance score much lower than a verbal score on a short form of the WISC shows some association with brain disorder. Using a difference equivalent to 25 points in IQ score terms, 13 out of 84 children with neuro-epileptic disorders had discrepancies as large as this or larger in favour of the verbal scale. This compared with 11 out of 147 in the control group. Thus, very large V – P discrepancies were almost twice as common in the brain-injured group.

However, a further cautionary note needs to be sounded. The comparison that has just been made relates to a group of all brain-injured children of a particular age range and a small control group drawn to represent the remaining 'normal' children. When the clinician meets a child in the clinic and discovers that the child has a verbal IQ some 25 points higher than his performance IQ, he cannot on the basis of the above data conclude that the child is twice as likely as not to belong to the brain-injured group. To draw such an inference would be to ignore the base-rate problem so ably discussed by *Meehl and Rosen* (1955).

Let us examine more closely what the above data really imply. 14% of the children with brain disorder have such a large discrepancy. (Note that this is the minority. 86% do not have the supposedly typical profile, and indeed about 5% have their performance score some 25 points greater than their verbal score.) But only 7.5% of the controls have a similar discrepancy. This means that if the controls are truly representative of the total population from which they were drawn at random, then there are some 550–800 of the 11,865 children who have such large discrepancies but who show no signs of brain injury. At a conservative estimate, therefore, the odds *against* a child with a (V–P) discrepancy of 25 points having brain injury are in the region of 500–13.

In summary, it is very difficult in psychometric terms to interpret differences between test scores. The tests themselves need to be reliable and valid, and one has to use sophisticated statistical techniques to evaluate the reliability of differences between scores in purely statistical terms. There is no guarantee that even statistically reliable differences will prove clinically significant particularly when the base rate of occurrence of the differences is examined in contrasting groups. Little wonder that psychometric testing is often undervalued – its practitioners have too often promised inappropriate results on the basis of inadequate empirical data. And yet, as I have argued earlier, I believe that such testing has an important but limited role in developmental assessment.

The Behavioural, Single-Case Study Approach

Is there then, an alternative approach to making a developmental psychological assessment of a child referred because of some hearing difficulty. I believe that there is, and that it is much more in keeping with the traditions of experimental psychology.

Many years ago, *Shapiro* (1951) outlined what he termed was an experimental approach to the investigation of individual cases. He has elaborated this view much more recently (*Shapiro,* 1970). Briefly, he argues that the best way to understand a psychological deficit is to find a way of measuring it and to bring that variable under experimental control; find out what, if anything, in the environment can be altered to bring about a concomitant change in the dependent variable of interest.

Over 20 years after this approach was expounded, it is being recognised as valuable in the investigation of children with learning disabilities. *Meichenbaum* (1976) calls his approach a 'cognitive-functional' approach, but acknowledges his intellectual debt to *Shapiro*.

More generally, the applied-behaviour-analysis approach adopts an experimental approach to individual cases (*Yule and Hemsley,* 1977). *Sulzbacher*

(1975) illustrates how their method of functional analysis can be brought to bear on the problems of the learning-disabled or hyperactive child. Like *Cohen* (1976) and *Ross* (1976), *Sulzbacher* argues that the first requirement is to pinpoint the behaviour that is causing concern. Get away from interpretive labels: return to the basic behaviour. Decide whether the behaviour complained of is causing a problem because it is present in excess or in deficit, and work out a treatment programme to remedy the situation. If you have made a current analysis of the problem, continuous monitoring should reveal changes in the behaviour in the desired direction. Failure allows one to exclude a particular hypothesis.

This approach is welcomed by many educationalists (*Bateman,* 1973). There is no time to discuss it more fully here, but let me illustrate the approach by quoting two relevant studies.

In one of the earliest published studies of the effects of behaviour modification techniques in the classroom, *Patterson et al.* (1965) increased the attending behaviour of a 10-year-old, brain-injured, retarded boy. After defining 'attending behaviour' in minute detail, observers recorded the boy's behaviour over a baseline period. Then, the child was provided with an earphone which signalled him every 10 sec that he did not display any of the behaviours incompatible with attending to his work. Over a 3 week treatment phase, the boy's non-attending dropped significantly. Later studies have been able to build on this pioneering research, and have been able to simplify the methods so that classroom teachers can implement the treatment without the use of complex apparatus or outside observers.

A second study will illustrate that one does not have to be a convert to behaviour modification to use the experimental methodology. As noted earlier, *Meichenbaum* (1976) and his colleagues have developed a number of cognitive strategies, based on the work of Luria, to teach self-control to overactive children. *Meichenbaum and Goodman* (1971) studied 3 groups of 5 children aged about 5 years. They were selected as 'impulsive' on their scores on the Matching Familiar Figures Test. None of the children improved their scores merely by being instructed not to hurry. One group were allowed to watch a model completing similar tasks. The model carried out a running commentary on his own performance, and then asked the children to do things as he had done them. The second group were additionally trained to produce self-instructions – they had to practice out loud telling themselves to be more careful, but in some detail. After training the first group (model only) took longer to make decisions, but did not reduce their error scores. The second group (modelling plus self-instruction training) both slowed down and reduced errors.

Thus, these two studies illustrate that relatively simple experimental techniques can be used to investigate phenomena such as 'poor attention' in the classroom or 'impulsiveness' in picture matching, and can bring such behaviours under experimental control. Clearly, such small-scale experiments have an enormous potential both in pinpointing deficits in individual cases and in providing techniques which can be used to ameliorate the associated problems.

Concluding Remarks

In many ways, I have ranged far and wide in this paper, largely because I did not find that the elegant title was clearly associated with any particular behavioural referrants – at least not once the concept of MBD was discarded in its present form. I hope that the resulting discussion is not too confusing. I believe that developmental assessment of the traditional, psychometric variety has still an important role in assessing children with learning disabilities. In particular, I think that it is only by studying clearly specified groups of children who share certain well-defined characteristics that much future progress will be made in this field.

However, psychometric assessment involves much more than merely 'giving tests'. I have tried to indicate some of the major pitfalls which exist in interpreting test results. We do have a wide range of useful tests at present, but they have to be used carefully and the results interpreted according to the highest standards of applied psychology.

Even so, test batteries rarely yield information directly relevant to teachers. Experimental investigations of single cases are much more relevant to meet such therapeutic needs. Thus, different professionals require different data, and there can be no such thing as a universally acceptable diagnosis.

Summary

Since I agree with *Ingram* (1973) when he says that ' "Minimal brain damage" is not a diagnosis; it is an escape from making one', how can I justify the title of this paper? It seems to me that MBD is a concept rather like 'dyslexia' – it may have been valuable in drawing attention to a heterogeneous group of developmental disorders, but its continuing usage is probably more harmful than helpful since (a) it assumes a homogeneous symptomatology, and (b) it implies a known aetiology – namely some form of brain damage or dysfunction. Neither of these implications is in line with research findings.

This is not to deny the existence of children with a wide variety of problems which appear to have a developmental/neurological component. Instead, there is a need to dispense with premature 'neurologizing', and return to a situation where the problems presented by the child are adequately *described* before they are interpreted. Such descriptions need to be in precise, behavioural terms. 'Signs', 'symptoms', 'delays' – all of them need to be operationally defined and means found of measuring them objectively.

At present, developmental psychological assessment is in a peculiar state. Assessments consist of a mixture of standardized tests – some with sound theoretical bases, others with no theoretical bases – and quasi-experimental techniques. Criterion referenced tasks exist alongside standardized instruments, and no two groups of workers agree on which form of assessment is most useful for which purpose. Too often, assessment is seen as an end in itself, and little thought is given to providing evidence which has implications for treatment as well as for diagnosis.

In this paper, I propose to review some of the procedures which are used in assessing those aspects of the MBD constellation which have received most attention – visuo-spatial problems; language delays, various forms of underachievement, clumsiness, hyperactivity, impulsivity, attention span and the like. I will argue that much better assessment tools are required. Just because 'neuropsychology' is an art form, that is no excuse for accepting sloppy assessment standards.

I will draw attention to two widely differing approaches to assessing neurological problems in children – (a) the 'battery' approach followed by such workers as *Reitan, Doehring* and *Rourke,* and (b) the behavioural, therapeutic approach followed by *Ross* and *Conners.*

The former group often discuss psychometric 'profiles', and I will draw attention to the intuitive attractiveness but empirical poverty of this approach. In particular, I will discuss two recurring problems: (i) the continuing use of WISC Verbal-Performance discrepancies in diagnosis despite the paucity of studies to support this procedure, and (ii) the effects of low base-rate of occurrence of a pathological condition on making predictions from any sign or index.

I am more attracted by the approach of the behavioural, interventionist group, but since so few studies have been undertaken in this model it is too early to draw conclusions from their findings. However, most clinicians would agree that any assessment which leads to better and more efficient treatment is *a priori* to be preferred.

I will finish by presenting some views on which forms of assessment I think should be developed as a matter of priority. These will include measures of language development and attention as well as 'hyperactivity'. However, as much effort should be put into refining concepts such as 'underachievement'. Finally, psychologists seem to have lost sight of measures such as reaction time and latency of response which seem to be potentially more subtle indices of neuro-developmental disorder.

References

Anthony, A.; Bogle, D.; Ingram, T.T.S., and McIsaac, M.W.: The Edinburgh articulation test (Churchill Livingstone, Edinburgh 1971).

Bandura, A.: Aggression. A social learning analysis (Prentice Hall, London 1973).

Bateman, B.D.: Educational implications of minimal brain dysfunction. Ann. N.Y. Acad. Sci. *205:* 245–250 (1973).

Becker, R.D.: The neurology of childhood learning disorders. The minimal brain dysfunction syndrome re-examined. Therap. Educ. *4:* 20–31 (1976).

Benton, A.L.: Minimal brain dysfunction from a neuropsychological point of view. Ann. N.Y. Acad. Sci. *205:* 29–37 (1973).

Berger, M.: The third revision of the Standford-Binet (Form L–M). Some methodological limitations and their practical implications. Bull. Br. psychol. Soc. *23:* 17 (1970).

Berger, M. and Yule, W.: Cognitive assessment in young children with language delay; in *Rutter and Martin* The child with delayed speech (Heinemann Medical, London 1972).

Berger, M.; Yule, W., and Rutter, M.: Attainment and adjustment in two geographical areas. II. The prevalence of specific reading retardation. Br. J. Psychiat. *126:* 510–519 (1975).

Block, J.; Block, J.H., and Harrington, D.M.: Some misgivings about the Matching Familiar Figures Test as a measure of reflection-impulsivity. Devl Psychol. *10:* 611–632 (1974).

Bortner, M.: Psychological deficit; in *Bortner* Evaluation and education of children with brain damage (Thomas, Springfield 1968).
Cohen, S.A.: Minimal brain dysfunction and practical matters such as teaching kids to read. Ann. N.Y. Acad. Sci. *205:* 251–261 (1973).
Cohen, S.A.: The fuzziness and the flab. Some solutions to research problems in learning disabilities. J. spec. Educ. *10:* 129 (1976).
Conners, C.K.: Psychological assessment of children with minimal brain dysfunction. Ann. N.Y. Acad. Sci. *205:* 283–302 (1973).
Doehring, D.G.: Patterns of impairment in specific reading disability. A neuropsychological investigation (Indiana University Press, Bloomington 1968).
Field, J.G.: Two types of tables for use with Wechsler's intelligence scales. J. clin. Psychol. *16:* 3 (1960).
Frostig, M.; Lefever, D.W., and Whittlesey, J.R.B.: The Marianne Frostig Developmental Test of Visual Perception Calif.: (Consulting Psychologists Press, Palo Alto 1964).
Halverson, C.F. and Waldrop, M.F.: The relations of mechanically recorded activity level to varieties of preschool play behavior. Child Dev. *44:* 678–681 (1973).
Hopkins, M.D.: An empirical analysis of the efficacy of the WISC in the diagnosis of organicity in children of normal intelligence. J. gen. Psychol. *105:* 163–172 (1964).
Ingram, T.T.S.: Soft signs (Annotation). Devl Med. Child Neurol. *15:* 527–529 (1973).
Kagan, J.: Reflection-impulsivity and reading ability in primary grade children. Child Dev. *36:* 609–628 (1965).
Kalverboer, A.F.: A neurobehavioural study in pre-school children (Heinemann Medical, London 1973).
Kassinove, H. and Summers, M.: The developmental attention test. A preliminary report of an objective test of attention. J. clin. Psychol. *24:* 76–78 (1968).
Kirk, S.A.; McCarthy, J.J., and Kirk, W.: The Illinois Test of Psycholinguistic Abilities (revised ed.) (Univ. Illinois, Institute for Research in Exceptional Children, Illinois 1968).
Klein, D.F. and Gittelman-Klein, R.: Problems in the diagnosis of minimal brain dysfunction in the hyperkinetic syndrome. Int. J. ment. Hlth *4:* 45–60 (1975).
Knights, R.M. and Bakker, D.J.: The neuropsychology of learning disorders. Theoretical approaches (University Park Press, Baltimore 1976).
Meehl, P.E. and Rosen, A.: Antecedent probability of the efficiency of psychometric signs, patterns or cutting scores. Psychol. Bull. *52:* 194–216 (1955).
Meichenbaum, D.: Cognitive functional approach to cognitive factors as determinants of learning disabilities; in *Knights and Bakker* The neuropsychology of learning disorders. Theoretical approaches (University Park Press, Baltimore 1976).
Meichenbaum, D.H. and Goodman, J.: Training impulsive children to talk to themselves. A means of developing self control. J. abnorm. Psychol. *77:* 115–126 (1971).
Mittler, P. and Ward, J.: The use of the Illinois Test of Psycholinguistic Abilities with English four-year-old children. A normative and factorial study. Br. J. educ. Psychol. *40:* 43 (1970).
Olson, A.V.: Factor analytic studies of the Frostig Developmental Test of Visual Perception. J. spec. Educ. *2:* 429 (1968).
Osgood, C.E.: A behavioristic analysis; in *Osgood* Contemporary approaches to cognition (MIT Press, Cambridge 1957).
Palermo, D.S.: Language acquisition; in *Reese and Lipsitt* Experimental child psychology (Academic Press, New York 1970).
Patterson, G.R. and Brodsky, G.: A behaviour modification programme for a child with multiple problem behaviour. J. child Psychol. Psychiat. *7:* 277–295 (1966).

Patterson, G.R.; Jones, R.; Whittier, J., and Wright, M.A.: A behaviour modification technique for the hyperactive child. Behav. Res. Ther. *2:* 217–226 (1965).

Payne, R.W. and Jones, H.G.: Statistics for the investigation of individual cases. J. clin. Psychol. *13:* 115–121 (1957).

Reitan, R.M. and Heineman, C.: Interactions of neurological deficits and emotional disturbances in children with learning disorders. Methods for their differential assessment; in *Hellmuth* Learning disorders, vol. 3 (Special Child Publications, Seattle 1957).

Reynell, J.K.: The Reynell Developmental Language Scales (NFER, Slough 1969).

Ross, A.O.: Psychological aspects of learning disabilities and reading disorders (McGraw-Hill, New York 1976).

Rourke, B.P.: Brain-behavior relationships in children with learning disabilities. Am. Psychol. *30:* 911–920 (1975).

Rourke, B.P.: Issues in neuropsychological assessment of children with learning disabilities. Can. psychol. Rev. *17:* 89 (1976).

Rutter, M.; Graham, P., and Yule, W.: A neuropsychiatric study in childhood (Heineman Medical, London 1970a).

Rutter, M.; Tizard, J., and Whitmore, K.: Education, health and behaviour (Longmans, London 1970b).

Rutter, M. and Yule, W.: The concept of specific reading retardation. J. Child Psychol. Psychiat. *16:* 181–197 (1975).

Sattler, J.M.: Assessment of children's intelligence (Saunders, Philadelphia 1974).

Shapiro, M.B.: An experimental approach to diagnostic psychological testing. J. ment. Sci. *97:* 748–764 (1951).

Shapiro, M.B.: Intensive assessment of the single case. An inductive-deductive approach; in *Mittler* Psychological assessment of mental and physical handicaps (Methuen, London 1970).

Sprague, R.L.; Barnes, K.R., and Werry, J.S.: Methylphenidate and thioridazine. Learning, reaction time, activity and classroom behavior in disturbed children. Am. J. Orthopsychiat. *40:* 615–628 (1970).

Staats, A.W.: Learning, language and cognition (Holt, Rinehart Winston, New York 1968).

Sulzbacher, S.I.: The learning-disabled or hyperactive child. Diagnosis and treatment. J. Am. med. Ass. *234:* 938–941 (1975).

Thorndike, R.L.: The concepts of over- and under-achievement (Bureau of publications, Teachers College, Columbia University, New York 1963).

Touwen, B.C.L. and Prechtl, H.F.R.: The neurological examination of the child with minor nervous dysfunction (Heinemann Medical, London 1970).

Wender, P.H.: The minimal brain dysfunction syndrome. Ann. Rev. Med. *26:* 45–62 (1975).

Yule, W.: Predicting reading ages on Neale's analysis of reading ability. Br. J. educ. Psychol. *37:* 252–255 (1967).

Yule, W.: Issues and problems in remedial education. Devl Med. Child Neurol. *18:* 675–682 (1976).

Yule, W. and Berger, M.: Communication, language and behaviour modification; in *Kiernan and Woodford* Behaviour modification with the severely retarded (Associated Scientific Publishers, Amsterdam 1975).

Yule, W. and Hemsley, D.: Single-case method in medical psychology; in *Rachman* Contributions to medical psychology. (Pergamon Press, Oxford 1977).

Dr. *W. Yule*, Senior Lecturer in Psychology, Institute of Psychiatry, Department of Psychology, De Crespigny Park, Denmark Hill, *London SE5 8AF* (England)

Adv. biol. Psychiat., vol. 1, pp. 55–67 (Karger, Basel 1978)

Minimal Brain Dysfunction and Minor Neurological Dysfunction

B.C.L. Touwen
Institut voor Ontwikkelingsneurologie, Academisch Ziekenhuis, Groningen

At first glance it may appear strange to put the terms 'Minimal Brain Dysfunction' and 'Minor Neurological Dysfunction' side by side. The term 'Minimal Brain Dysfunction' is used to identify children with behaviour and/or learning problems which are assumed to be connected with 'Minor Neurological Dysfunction'. The veracity of this assumption, however, can be queried, and the literature on MBD certainly is not unequivocal on this point, neither pro nor contra (see *Kalverboer* in this volume). There is no doubt that children with behavioural and/or learning difficulties that can be subsumed under the heading MBD exist. Children with signs of minor neurological dysfunction exist as well, but they do not necessarily have behavioural difficulties.

Until further notice the present author chooses to regard MBD solely as a behavioural syndrome with a complex aetiology, a view expressed by *Birch* in 1964. Beside MBD and partly overlapping with it, MND may exist. In this connotation MND is a sign (or rather a number of signs) of neurological impairment, found on neurological investigation.

The Neurological Investigation

A neurological investigation is carried out to confirm any suspected impairment of the nervous system which manifests itself in the neurological condition of the patient. I emphasize the word 'neurological' in order to make clear that we are concerned with those elements of behaviour which can be evaluated with the help of neurological indices such as posture, motility and more specific reactions and responses. When one or more of these indices are found to be deviant, i.e., different from what is found in the majority of healthy individuals, then we are dealing with neurological impairment, which can be called 'major' or 'minor'. Such impairment of the nervous system may or may not be accompanied by disturbances in complex behaviour, which are commonly called 'behavioural difficulties'. There are two other important points. Firstly, during childhood only a developmental neurological investigation can be considered appropriate. This neurological technique involves taking full account of the properties of the developing nervous system. An essential characteristic of the technique is the age-specificity both in the content of the procedure and of the manipulations. It is then possible to identify neurological deviations which may only occur during development and which may be overlooked when the traditional adult techniques are used. Secondly, the technique should be able to detect both major and minor neurological deviations. This point is important, when the neurological condition of patients with behavioural difficulties is examined, in order to find out whether there may be a relationship between neurology and behaviour.

Minor and Major Neurological Impairment

What is meant by 'major' and 'minor' neurological impairment in this context? We are concerned with a *'major' neurological impairment* when a child's abilities in daily behaviour are grossly impaired, which is the case with patients suffering from cerebral palsy. The neurological examination is then used to make a proper diagnosis of the disturbance which underlies the functional impairment; it is also needed to evaluate those functions which are still preserved. This latter aim is important for treatment purposes, for instance, physiotherapy in patients with cerebral palsy.

The term 'minor' neurological impairment covers two categories of patients: firstly, there are the patients who have a slight functional handicap, which is not very conspicuous and which does not incapacitate them in their daily life. However, the neurological examination reveals definite signs, and the problems of the patient can be associated with the neurological findings. In such cases the term *'minimal' cerebral palsy* is often used; this is a functional term, which does not claim a direct relationship between the degree of the neurological impairment and the extent of the structural brain lesion. In general the neurological findings can be interpreted in a comparable way to the findings in cases of (major) cerebral palsy.

The second category labeled 'minor' neurological impairment, consists of patients who do not give evidence of any functional impairment which can be related directly to neurological dysfunction. Usually the patient's problems do not suggest a neurological impairment as is the case in (minimal) cerebral palsy, and the patient is usually not primarily referred to a neurologist. Patients may be somewhat clumsy or show unusual movement patterns or a lot of movements which are more or less inadequate, but not necessarily in all cases. Such motor behaviour, if present, is hardly ever considered to be the result of a neurological impairment. On thorough and comprehensive neurological examination (*Touwen and Prechtl,* 1970), however, signs of neurological dysfunction can be demonstrated which may be of slight intensity but which are nevertheless consistently present. It is often impossible to arrange them into a recognizable clinical pattern with a clear diagnostic label, but they must be interpreted as reflecting a neurological dysfunction because they are absent in the majority of healthy normal children. Again a direct relationship between the degree of neurological dysfunction and the extent of structural damage to the brain cannot be postulated (*Windle,* 1969; *Prechtl,* 1973). Moreover, the clinical significance of the neurological findings is often unclear. The presence of such slight deviations can be the first sign of a progressive disease but this is rarely the case.

Hard and Soft Signs

Minor signs are often referred to as 'soft signs', due to problems of either elicitation, replication or interpretation. Thus, the term 'soft sign' implies doubt about its usefulness for neurological diagnosis, in contrast to 'hard signs'. However, the argument that elicitation and replication are difficult to achieve is not valid. A sign is not a neurological sign when it cannot be elicited properly or be replicated by the same or a different examiner (*Rutter et al.*, 1970).

The fact that the interpretation of a sign cannot be made does not imply that it is a 'soft' sign. The clinical significance of a sign, 'soft' or 'hard', is often difficult to understand, and often manifold. In the case of 'hard' signs, this difficulty can be illustrated by, e.g., the Babinski response which often can only be interpreted tentatively. Thus the nomenclature 'soft' or 'equivocal' for minor neurological findings should be discarded: a sign is a sign, although we may not know what it means.

Optimality

As stated above the neurological signs often cannot be grouped into recognizable clinical patterns. A solution is to apply *Prechtl*'s (1968) optimality concept, which was developed originally to describe the obstetric history and the neurological condition of a newborn infant quantitatively. For all neurological items of the assessment, an optimal range is defined. This means that those performances are defined which must be considered perfect. The optimal ranges for the items can be defined on the basis of theoretical considerations and clinical experience. Population norms are not needed as optimality is not identical with 'normality'. In the case of standing upright for instance, the

Table I. Groups of items for several artificially distinguished subsystems of the nervous system used for a neurological profile

1 Sensorimotor apparatus
Resistance to passive movement
Muscle power
Range of movements
Muscle consistency
Knee jerk
Ankle jerk
Threshold muscle reflexes legs
Biceps reflex
Triceps reflex
Threshold muscle reflexes arms
Abdominal skin reflex
Foot sole reflex
Other exteroceptive reflexes big toe

2 Posture
Sitting, general
Feet, sitting
Standing, general
Legs, standing
Feet, standing
Extended arms, standing
Walking
Lying in prone and supine

3 Balance of trunk
Response to push, standing
Following object with eyes and head
Romberg
Rebound phenomenon
Walking on a straight line

4 Co-ordination of the extremities
Fingertip–nose test
Diadochokinesis
Knee–heel test
Kicking against hand
Fingertip touching test

5 Fine manipulative ability
Finger-opposition test
Follow-a-finger test
Circle test

6 (Dys)kinesia
Choreiform movements distal
Choreiform movements proximal
Choreiform movements during spontaneous behaviour
Athetotiform movements

7 Gross motor functions
Heel–toe gait
Walking on tiptoe
Walking on heels
Standing on one leg
Hopping on one leg
Rising into sitting

8 Quality of motility

Speed Smoothness Adequacy	small motor movement
Speed Smoothness Adequacy	gross motor movement

9 Associated movements
M.O.F.S.
Mirror movement diadochokinesis
A.m. tiptoe
A.m. heels
A.m. index-thumb grasp

10 Visual system
Position of the eyes
Directional nystagmus
Position nystagmus
Optokinetic nystagmus
Pursuit movements of the eyes
Visual fields
Fundoscopy

For technique and scoring, see *Touwen and Prechtl* (1970).

examiner knows that symmetry is optimal, and asymmetry is non-optimal, and in the case of reflexes such as the patellar tendon reflex a medium intensity of the reflex can be considered optimal compared with a low and a high intensity. This last example illustrates that optimality overlaps normality. It stands to reason, however, that age-specificity is essential: at different ages different responses can be regarded as optimal. Adding up the total number of optimal performances results in an optimality score which measures the integrity of the nervous system quantitatively, i.e., by comparison with the potential maximum optimality score. This method is based on the conception that a decreasing amount of optimal performances reflects an increasing functional impairment of the brain. At the same time a neurological sign with definite clinical significance will never occur without other signs of non-optimality being present.

It is obvious that an optimality score need only be estimated when no traditional diagnosis can be made: it enables the examiner to quantify and describe his concern about a child when it cannot be done adequately by any other means.

The Neurological Profile

The optimality score should be used in combination with the original data, because it gives a *quantification* and not a specific *qualification* of the nervous integrity of a child. For a more differentiated evaluation of the child's neurological condition, the neurological items are placed into groups, representing artificially distinguished subsystems of the nervous system, such as sensorimotor, posture, coordination, etc. (table I). For each group the number of optimal performances is counted which provides a neurological profile (*Touwen and Kalverboer,* 1973). An example is given in figure 1 which shows a child with an optimal sensorimotor and posture subsystem, while trunk co-ordination, co-ordination of the extremities and the items describing fine manipulative ability are non-optimal. Also, gross motor functions such as hopping and standing on one leg are non-optimal and there is a dyskinesia of the choreiform type. At the same time, 'post' or 'propter', the child's motility does not appear to be within optimal limits.

It must be emphasized that a profile can only be drawn up after a comprehensive neurological examination. The profile enables the examiner to screen rapidly in which functional areas the child is impaired, while a comparison with the original data tells him what exactly is wrong with this particular child. This can be informative from two points of view. Firstly, it is possible to discern children with particular dysfunctions, e.g. coordination troubles or dyskinesias, or combinations, which may be useful for research into specific

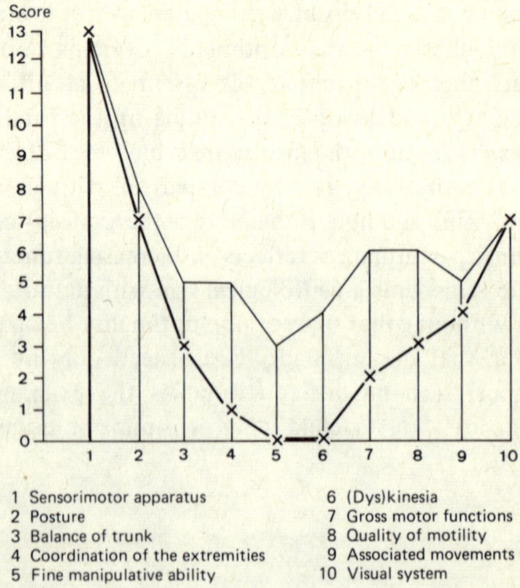

Fig. 1. An example of a neurological profile. This 6-year-old boy shows low optimality scores in the groups 3, 4, 5 and 6. The low scores in 7 and 8 can be considered as a result. The quality of the non-optimal performances must be traced back on the original examination protocol. Patient R.P., male, 6 years.

relationships between neurological dysfunctions and behaviour. Secondly, it may suggest a specific treatment of neurological dysfunction, for instance in the case of co-ordination difficulties or fine manipulative difficulties.

Minor Neurological Dysfunction

Up till now I have avoided the use of the term 'minor neurological dysfunction'. It was purposely done as the term could be interpreted as a specific diagnosis. However, 'minor neurological dysfunction' is only a general term, referring to a group of various neurological conditions which have one thing in common, namely, that the manifested neurological impairment is slight and inconspicuous. Proper diagnoses of minor neurological dysfunction are usually descriptive. They describe, for instance, co-ordination difficulties or manipulative disabilities, or dyskinesias such as choreiform movements. 'Minor neurological dysfunction' should be regarded as a term like 'cerebral palsy', being very unspecific and requiring further exploration of what is really wrong with the patient.

Minimal Brain Dysfunction

What is the significance of the neurological findings where one is concerned with the MBD issue? As stated above, 'minor neurological dysfunction' is a general term which covers a variety of diagnoses of slight neurological impairment. 'Minimal brain dysfunction' is also a general term; it is used for various conditions which are usually delineated insufficiently and not diagnosed properly. Actually, the term MBD only refers to a group of deviant behavioural symptoms, which tend to concur but which may have quite different aetiologies, varying from a socio-environmental or educational, to an emotional or even a genetic causation.

There may be also a neurological impairment. It is remarkable that such impairment is usually 'minor' and rarely 'major'. It is of little help to use the name MBD as a diagnosis before the behavioural problems and their aetiology are properly analysed. MBD is not a diagnosis, and the use of the term MBD implies that diagnostic procedures have to start. Among these procedures the neurological investigation is of primary importance because there are children with behavioural problems who may be neurologically impaired. It is hardly wise to pose the question: should one look for a relationship between MBD and MND? It is, however, sensible to consider a (causal) relationship between behavioural difficulties and neurological impairment for children who show both sets of symptoms.

Neurological Impairment and Behaviour

Does neurological impairment play a role in the genesis of behavioural difficulties apart from what is known about major dysfunctions like frontal lobe tumours or epilepsy? It is sometimes possible to discern a link between specific neurological findings and behavioural disturbances. Take for instance an inattentive child with a rather low intelligence level, who lives with his large lower-middle class family in a small flat and whose father, unhappily, is a quick-tempered man while his mother suffers from morning moods. He has also slight co-ordination difficulties. It is not unlikely that for his family this child is a continuous source of tension because of his clumsy motility. Again and again he upsets his cup of milk on the breakfast table, again and again he stumbles against the chairs in the crowded living room. The child's behaviour together with the reaction of the family to his behaviour may result in a serious behavioural syndrome. It is evident that in this case the neurological dysfunction is not the sole cause for the behavioural difficulties; still it plays an important part in its aetiology. Thus, one might contend that there is a relationship. It is important to discern this relationship, as it may suggest which treatments would be suitable. In the above case, for example, physiotherapy for the co-ordination problems combined with other treatments, such as family therapy, may help to reduce the difficulties.

Another hypothesis might be derived about the relation between neurological dysfunction and behavioural disturbances in a group of children who are said to suffer from MBD. Call it the paradox of disturbed behaviour in children with MND. Elsewhere, I have pointed out that variability is an essential characteristic of healthy neurological functioning (*Touwen,* 1976). In general, one has to distinguish between variations of normal functioning which are characteristic of the healthy brain, based on the extensive properties of the nervous system, and pathological motor patterns, which may give the impression of variability, whereas they are distortions of normal functioning. The so-called normal variability has at least two aspects. In the first place a pre-set goal – for instance, standing up, walking, grasping – can be reached along various ways, the brain using various strategies at various times. The saying: 'There are many roads which lead to Rome' might be applied here. This type of variability reflects the adaptability of the brain which enables the individual to cope with the environmental demands in various ways, in accordance with immediate requirements. Secondly, many neurological items have an easily recognizable response-pattern, and are therefore used in a neurological examination, but when looked at in detail, they appear to have a high degree of intra-individual variability (e.g. reactions and responses). In a healthy person, hopping reactions (on tilting) or withdrawal reactions to a pin prick of the footsole are never identical from one trial to the other, although the outcomes may be directly comparable. That is to say: although such neural functions may seem to be stereotyped, their stereotypy is limited.

One characteristic of either minor or major neurological dysfunction is a diminution of both aspects of variability. In the first place the possibility of choosing between various strategies is diminished, in other words many of the roads to Rome are closed. This may lead to stereotyped motor performances, and a lack of adaptability. For example, the gait of a diplegic patient is stereotyped compared with that of a normal child. This stereotyped pattern has a distorted appearance compared with normal walking patterns. Still it is much less variable, and it has fewer possibilities of adaptation to changing environmental conditions. The same can be said of, e.g., an ataxic gait in the case of cerebellar impairment. Here also the motor pattern is distorted, its result is often unpredictable (it is difficult to predict when the patient will fall down), yet compared to the variability of gait of a normal person, there is an increase of stereotypy.

In the second place, in cases of brain impairment, stimulus-response relationships, e.g., reflexes and reactions, are far more fixed than is the case in normal individuals. A withdrawal reaction in a brain-damaged patient shows an evidently stronger stereotypy compared with for instance the withdrawal reaction of a healthy child.

Paradoxically many children with behavioural problems as described in the MBD syndrome show many aspects of behaviour which are said to be extremely variable and unpredictable. They react to the demands put upon them by their environment in an unexpected and often exaggerated way.

Thus, on the one hand there is an increase of stereotypy as a result of a diminished variability of the nervous system due to neurological dysfunction and on the other hand there is this irregular, unpredictable and unusual behaviour. This apparent contradiction may be solved in accordance with the theory proposed by *Popper* (1972). In *Popper*'s view problem solving should occur by way of trial and error elimination. During this process hypotheses are tested and then re-formulated taking into account the errors which became evident during the test trials. Thus, the elimination of the errors leads to a refinement of the hypothesis. This theory can be usefully applied in the field of neurology. During development the brain continually receives messages which must be decoded and tested on their usefulness. According to *Popper* this is done in the 'problem solving' way: based on innate dispositions actions are 'selected', which turn out to be right or wrong; in the latter case there is a process of error elimination, and so on and so forth until the best possible solution in the particular situation is arrived at. In this way the nervous system 'learns' to cope with the ever-changing demands of the environment. In the healthy child the brain will 'learn' different solutions in various situations. Moreover, the healthy nervous system has at its disposal a number of modes of operation to reach required ends, which means that a problem can be solved in various ways. This is what I call the variability of the healthy brain, which provides the basis for adaptive responses in specific contexts. During normal development the problem solving process goes on continually and automatically, resulting in (more or less) well-adapted behaviour.

In the case of neurological dysfunction, however, the brain is not so well equipped to adapt itself to the continually changing demands of the environment. Now four things may happen: Firstly, the nervous system may not be able to follow various modes of operation in different situations: it follows one and the same mode for solving a variety of problems, which results in stereotyped and often inadequate behaviour.

An extreme example of this phenomenon are temper tantrums, a primitive form of coping with otherwise unsolvable problems. As we know in children with behavioural difficulties, temper tantrums often occur without any apparent immediate cause. The parent often does not know when to expect them, so that the impression is gained of a child with unpredictable behaviour.

Secondly, in children with neurological dysfunction the process of trial and error elimination may last much longer than in normal children. Due to a deficiency of the 'hardware' of the nervous system the best program to be used with regard to the problem in question is not easily found, and many trials have to be made. But in the meantime the childs grows older, and his brain attains a higher degree of structural complexity. This may explain part of the pseudo-infantile behaviour of some children with behavioural difficulties. Although at first glance their behaviour appears to belong to a younger age it is still partly in accordance with the more complex brain specific for their age. It can therefore not be called retarded behaviour, but rather age-inadequate and unusual. Thirdly, in the case of neurological dysfunction the brain may not be able to find the proper solution for its task requirements as a result of its limited potentiality. It has to take refuge in less adequate or unusual modes of operation in order to meet the demands of the environment. One may call this 'substitution', but it is often a deficient substitution. Finally, there may remain errors notwithstanding the trial and error elimination process, either because the brain does not recognize them as errors, or because the brain is not able to eliminate them. From a morphological standpoint one may contend that the inadequate or even unsuccessful modes of operation are based in part on structural defects or perhaps on a 'wrong' re-modeling in the damaged brain (see *Prechtl,* this volume). However this may be, the use of such modes may explain part of the strange, often inadequate and unpredictable reactions of some children with behavioural difficulties. The reactions themselves may be stereotyped in relation to the environmental event(s) by which they are provoked, but their distribution over time may be unpredictable.

The four possibilities are depicted in figure 2. It has to be borne in mind that the possibilities are not mutually exclusive. Obviously there is a wide overlap and an intricate relationship between them.

I will emphasize the point that this hypothesis does not explain the MBD syndrome. It may merely explain part of the behaviour of neurologically impaired children who show a behavioural symptomatology as described under the heading MBD. Naturally, inappropriate reactions of the environment to the child's adaptive attempts will serve to reinforce the inadequate behavioural patterns to a large extent. Nevertheless, this hypothesis about a possible relation between neurological impairment and behavioural difficulties appears to suggest a type of treatment, which would mainly consist of ways in which to help the child with his trial and error elimination in specific situations.

In accordance with this hypothesis we try to treat children who are labeled MBD children, and who cannot be tolerated any longer by their families. The treatment consists of an efficient but simple programming of the daily occupa-

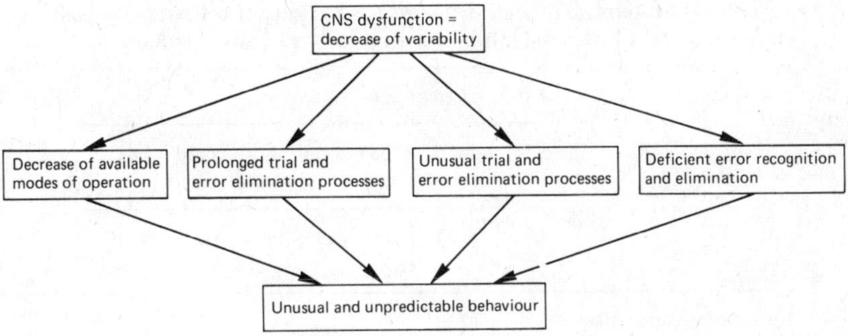

Fig. 2. The paradox of disturbed behaviour in children with minor neurological dysfunction.

tions, the avoidance of sudden and unexpected environmental stimuli, and a careful and extensive informing of the child about what he is expected to do and what he is going to experience. A painstaking observation of the child's behaviour, especially of his behavioural disturbances, is carried out concurrently, and fed back into the programming of his daily life, both in the institute and home settings.

We have recently analysed some pilot study[1] data which suggests that in general MBD children with evidence of MND react favourably to this type of treatment, while children with MBD symptomatology without MND or with an evident other aetiology, such as early affective neglect or severe neuroticism, react less favourably. In table II, the findings are summarized. Broad categories of mental retardation, early affective neglect, disruptive environment, and neuroticism are used to describe possible and recognizable aetiologies of the behavioural difficulties. The results are divided into 'short-term' effects of the treatment, meaning improvement during the stay in the institute (averaging 1–2 years), and 'long-term' effects defined as the outcome at a follow-up when the children had been at least 1 year at home. As during their stay in the institute the children spent all weekends (from Friday night till Sunday night) and all holidays at home, the short-term effects of the treatment do not merely denote the behavioural improvement in the institute, but also in the home environment. The effect is graded positive when the parents had no complaints, moderate when there were some difficulties, but not severe enough to warrant readmission to any institute, and negative when the behavioural difficulties remained so severe that the child could not be tolerated at home. An essential point in the

[1] This pilot study was carried out in 'Huize Groenendaal', Helper Haven, Groningen (Director: Dr. *K. Heslinga*) in co-operation with *P. de Berg* (pedagogue) and *J.H. van der Meulen* (psychologist).

Table II. Short-term (ST) and long-term (LT) results of behavioural treatment of 34 children (30 M; 4 F) labeled MBD for age range 5–12 years ($\bar{X}$ = 8.0 years)

Aetiology	Effect of treatment						Total
	ST: good	good	good	moderate	moderate	bad	
	LT: good	moderate	bad	moderate	bad	bad	
No aetiology evident	11						11
Mental retardation	2[1]	1		1	1	1[2]	6
Early affective neglect		1					1
Disruptive environment		2					2
Neuroticism		1					1
2 + 3 + 4					2[3]		2
3 + 4		1	1	1	1	1[2,4]	5
3 + 5						1[2]	1
3 + 4 + 5			2[5]	1	2		5
Total	13	6	3	3	6	3	34

[1] Borderline cases for mental retardation (1 girl and 1 boy).
[2] No MND.
[3] 1 girl without MND, 1 boy with MND.
[4] Girl.
[5] 1 girl, 1 boy.

treatment is that in no instance was any psychopharmacological treatment administered.

Although the admission criteria did not include neurological dysfunction, but were based on the well-known symptomatology of MBD behaviour, there were only 4 children without MND. Without exception these children did not profit from the treatment. Furthermore, it is clear from the table that an increase in the complexity of the aetiology appears to be related with a decrease of the efficiency of the treatment, especially with regard to the long-term results.

It should be borne in mind that these tabulated results represent preliminary findings. A major focus in the future progress of this study will be an operational refinement of the global diagnostic categories.

The possibility to distinguish the various results of the treatment support the view that MBD is only a vaguely delineated syndrome which should be properly diagnosed. I hope to have made it clear that during the process of diagnosing the developmental neurological investigation plays an important role.

Summary

MBD may be called a syndrome, but it is not an entity. It certainly means to describe a set of behavioural problems. Its aetiology may consist of various factors, including minor neurological impairment, but the role of minor neurological dysfunction in the aetiology of MBD behaviour often is not clear at all. The present paper pleads for a strict distinction between neurological and 'behavioural' investigation and diagnosis. For the neurological diagnosis the optimality score and the neurological profile are forwarded as suitable means if a traditional diagnosis cannot be made. A warning is given against the use of the term 'soft signs'.

In the second half of the paper a hypothesis, based on *Popper*'s problem-solving theory, is formulated in order to account for part of the MBD behaviour in patients with minor neurological dysfunction. This hypothesis has been applied for treatment of the behavioural problems. Preliminary results are presented.

References

Birch, H.G.: Brain damage in children. The biological and social aspects (Williams & Wilkins, Baltimore 1964).

Popper, K.R.: Objective knowledge. An evolutionary approach (Clarendon Press, Oxford 1972, reprinted edition 1975).

Prechtl, H.F.R.: Neurological findings in newborn infants after pre- and paranatal complications; in *Jonxis, Visser and Troelstra* Aspects of praematurity and dysmaturity. Nutricia Symposium, Leiden 1968, pp. 303–321.

Prechtl, H.F.R.: Das leicht hirn-geschädigte Kind. Theoretische Überlegungen zu einem praktischen Problem; in *Rümke, Boeke and van Dijk* Van kinderanalyse tot Y-chromosoom, pp. 282–305 (Van Loghum Slaterus, Deventer 1973).

Rutter, M.; Graham, P., and Yule, W.: A neuropsychiatric study in childhood. Clin. Dev. Med., No. 35/36 (Heinemann, London 1970).

Touwen, B.C.L.: Neurological development in infancy. Clin. Dev. Med., No. 58 (Heinemann, London 1976).

Touwen, B.C.L. and Kalverboer, A.F.: Neurologic and behavioral assessment of children with 'Minimal Brain Dysfunction'; in *Walzer and Wolff* Minimal cerebral dysfunction in children. Semin. Psychiat. *5:* 79–94 (1973).

Touwen, B.C.L. and Prechtl, H.F.R.: The neurological examination of the child with minor nervous dysfunction. Clin. Dev. Med., No. 38 (Heinemann, London 1970).

Windle, W.F.: Asphyxial damage at birth, with reference to the minimally affected child; in Perinatal factors affecting human development. Proceedings of the Special Session, 8th Meeting PAHO Advisory Committee on Medical Research, Scientif. Publication No. 185 (1969).

Dr. *B.C.L. Touwen,* Instituut voor Ontwikkelingsneurologie, Academisch Ziekenhuis, Oostersingel 59, *Groningen* (The Netherlands)

Adv. biol. Psychiat., vol. 1, pp. 68–83 (Karger, Basel 1978)

The Influence of Drugs on Minimal Brain Dysfunction

K. Pyck and P. Baines

Department of Brain and Behaviour, Child Psychiatry Unit, University Hospital Gasthuisberg, University of Leuven, Leuven

An enormous amount of literature has been published in the last 10 years about the MBD syndrome, but a clear and coherent psychopathological explanation has yet to be developed; neither is there a global psychiatric approach to diagnosis and treatment.

Pharmacological research, however, has an important role to play in the investigation of MBD, and we would like to review recent literature on this subject.

The first part of this article will describe the importance of pharmacological research, as part of the psychopathological and psychiatric investigation of MBD. In the second part the different types of drugs used in the MBD syndrome will be reviewed. The third part will describe the contribution pharmacological research can make to the knowledge of the MBD syndrome. In the last part of this review practical conclusions which can be used in the treatment of MBD children will be proposed.

The Role of Pharmacological Research in the Investigation of Psychiatric Disorders in Childhood

(a) Once a competent clinician has described a syndrome, psychopathological research will try to answer the following fundamental questions:

What is the exact description of this syndrome, and can it eventually be divided into separate subunits? What are the etiological factors and what are the pathogenetical mechanisms? What is the prognosis?

(b) Child psychiatry or clinical practice will try to answer the following practical questions:

Which diagnostic methods can be used, and which differential diagnosis must be made? What type of therapy is indicated, and what effect does this therapy have? Are there any preventive measures?

The answers to these questions require intensive research, and will be all the harder to find, if the syndrome is not precisely described, and if many etiological factors can be supposed to have a cumulative effect, and if secondary effects such as environmental factors are complex. The problem becomes even more complicated when causes and effects can be biological, psychological and social.

In answering these questions six stages should be examined, using an index population which complies with the initial clinical description (*Cantwell,* 1975).

(1) Clinical description. Careful clinical description of the behaviour problem; detailed, systematic, yet flexible questioning of parents; reliable information from the school; factors that may affect the clinical picture (age, sex, race, social class, etc.).

(2) Physical and neurological factors. Systematic and neurological examination, with evaluation of neurodevelopmental abnormalities.

(3) Laboratory studies. Blood, urine, spinal fluid, etc.; EEG, neurophysiological, neuroradiological exploration, etc.; neuropsychological investigation.

(4) Family studies. Studies of the prevalence and types of psychiatric disorders; studies of the relationships and interactions occurring between the members of a family.

(5) Natural history studies. Prospective and retrospective follow-up studies of the index population.

(6) Treatment studies, such as biological, psychological and educational.

Marked differences in response to adequate trials of the same treatment can be considered as evidence that the original group children did not form a homogeneous group.

The six stages of investigation should be made on the same index population and the results should be mutually compared before a coherent hypothesis can be formulated.

(c) Pharmacological research concerning clinical syndromes becomes especially important if it can differentiate subgroups, or if this research clarifies etiological or pathogenetic mechanisms, as has been the case in phenylketonuria. Both lines of research in MBD are promising but our actual knowledge is still very hypothetical, as the many contradictory research articles and clinical experience clearly demonstrate. It seems to us that this is because the problem is extremely complex, with continuous interaction between genetic factors and possible brain damage on one hand, and psychological, sociological and educational factors on the other.

All these factors can influence etiology and pathogenesis, prognosis and therapy. Therefore, definitive answers will only be found in a coordinated multidisciplinary approach.

Table I. Pharmaca used in the treatment of MBD children

1 Psychostimulant drugs	4 Lead chelation
2 Tricyclic antidepressants	Penicillamine
Imipramine	CA – EDTA
3 Major tranquillizers	5 Minor tranquillizers
Chlorpromazine (Largactil)	6 TRH
Thioridorazine (Melleril)	7 Lithium
Haloperidol (Haldol)	8 Antiepileptic drugs
	9 Nootropic drugs (Encefabol, Nootropil)

Table II. Psychostimulant drugs used in the treatment of MBD children

Psychostimulant drugs	Daily, mg
1 Dextroamfetamine (Dexedrine)	5–20
2 Methylphenidate (Ritalin)	10–40
3 Magnesium pemoline (Cylert, Stimul)	37.5–75
4 Caffeine	200–300
5 Levoamfetamine (Cydril)	7–30
6 Fenetyllin (Captagon)	25–40

Drug Therapy of MBD Children

Many different drugs have been used in the treatment of MBD children (table I), but we feel that the stimulant drugs merit most attention (table II) in our review. These drugs have been intensively studied in the last 10 years, and are extensively prescribed in the USA. About 2% of all elementary school children, i.e. 300,000–400,000 children, receive prescribed stimulant drugs (*Safer and Allen,* 1976). The National Institute of Mental Health estimated that approximately 4,000,000 hyperactive children could benefit from drugs (*Ross and Ross,* 1976). This subject has become highly controversial: *Wender* (1971), one of the most fervent defenders of drug therapy wrote that, 'The MBD syndrome is extremely common, being probably the most common single diagnostic entity seen in child guidance clinics. The treatment of choice in virtually all instances consists first of medication, second of counseling, and last of "psychotherapy".'

He modified his attitude slightly in 1974, when he said: 'A number of pharmacological and social therapies have been employed. The most dramatically effective, at least on a short-term basis, has been pharmacological. MBD children often respond dramatically to treatment with stimulant medication. It is this fact which has prompted so much controversy over the disorder and its treatment. If MBD children had had the wisdom and foresight to respond to

Lithium, their treatment would have avoided much moralistic invective from – Mirabile dictu – the far left and the far right' (*Wender,* 1974).

Sroufe (1975) however, in his review of drug therapy of children with behaviour problems, contests the frequency of drug treatment: 'Existing information concerning the effects of stimulant drugs on cognitive development, the persistence of behavioral effects, and the long-term physical and psychological consequences of these drugs is simply too limited to justify the current level of drug treatment.'

Psychostimulant Drugs

Methylphenidate and Dextroamphetamine

At present, two stimulants, methylfenidate (Ritalin) and dextroamphetamine (dexedrine) are the most widely used drugs for the pharmacological treatment of hyperactivity. Most research also concerns these two drugs.

The primary indication for stimulant drug treatment is hyperkinesis and short attention span; it appears that the more hyperactive the child is, the better the clinical response will be. Nonhyperactive, learning-impaired children do not show any improvement after stimulant medication. The clinical response to stimulant drugs is as follows: 30–50% show a dramatic improvement, such as less classroom restlessness, increased attention span, increased academic work output and accuracy, and improved emotional and social behavior patterns; the child becomes happier, more motivated and more successful. His social and emotional relationships improve, 20–40% show a moderate improvement, and 5–10% become worse, more erratic and irritable (*Ross and Ross,* 1976; *Safer and Allen,* 1976).

Most studies are of the double-blind crossover type, and most analyze the effect of a drug during a relatively short time (2–4 weeks). We feel this is too short, and this is one of the main criticisms of pharmacological research.

Overall research data can be summarised as follows: These stimulant drugs essentially effect activity during psychological testing, and they have much less effect in totally 'free' situations as play at school or at home (*Ellis et al.,* 1974). On attention or vigilance, such as the continuous performance test, hyperactive children show notable performance improvements after stimulant drugs. When compared to placebo takers, the children taking stimulants show decreased seat movements, fewer errors and fewer omissions (*Sprague et al.,* 1970; *Sykes et al.,* 1972).

Hyperactive children on stimulants also frequently show improved ability in fine motor performance tests and perceptual discrimination tests. These reflect improved visual motor skills, less impulsivity, better visual and auditory discrimination, and better short-term learning skills (*Conners,* 1971). Improvement in intelligence test performance has been consistently demonstrated on the Performance Scale of WISC, the Porteus Maze IQ score, and the Goudenough Draw-A-Man Test; the verbal IQ of WISC occasionally improves. However, these findings should not be interpreted as evidence that intelligence or learning ability can be increased with drug intervention; it is generally agreed that improvement in performance is a function of increased motivation and attention, which are of critical importance in test situations (*Conners,* 1972).

We studied the effect of Ritaline versus a placebo in a pilot study (*Pyck,* 1975): this was a double-blind crossover study of 45 children with hyperactivity syndrome. There were statistically significant differences in the teacher's rating scale for hyperkinetic behavior (1%), the educators' rating scale (5%), the Bender visual motor gestalt test, the revised Benton visual motor gestalt test, the revised Benton visual retention test, the Rey test, and in a screening test for neuromotor dysfunction (Hendrickx).

The short-term effects of stimulant medication are relatively well known, they are usually temporary, lasting not more than a week, and are usually minor. From 25 to 50% of children on stimulant drugs initially experience an appetite decrease, more so with dexedrine than with ritaline; if daily use is continued this becomes less obvious. Insomnia can occur if a noon or afternoon dose of stimulants is given. During the 1st week and occasionally during the 2nd, about 15% of children given stimulants complain of one of the following: headaches, vomiting, moodiness or a tendency to cry; we have usually seen this in mentally retarded hyperkinetic children. In some children pallor and a decrease in skin temperature of the face can occur with higher doses of stimulants; dyskinetic episodes and more recently tics (*Denckla et al.,* 1976) have been described, but they are also very rare (1% of treated children). It is also important to note that hyperkinetic children on stimulants do not become high or euphoric; should hyperactive children experience a notable mood change on stimulants, it is usually a temporary phase of depressive irritability, an occasional but infrequent side effect.

There have been few studies so far on the addictive risks of stimulants, but these do not show that this is a real danger. We would like to mention the long-term follow-up study of *Beck et al.* (1975), who found no correlation between the use of methylfenidate as a child and later drug abuse in adolescence. Compared to a control group, there were even significantly less drug addicts: only 2 out of 30 occasionally smoked marihuana, compared to a total of 8 in the controls (3 occasional users and 3 habitual users of marihuana, 1 occasional heroin user and 1 hashish user). Larger population studies are obviously needed.

Other Stimulant Drugs

Magnesium pemoline (tradename: Cylert or Stimul), is a newer stimulant drug, that has only recently been subjected to intensive research. *Conners et al.* (1972) compared the effect of pemoline, dexedrine and a placebo on 84 hyperactive children aged from 6 to 12 years. The ratings consistently showed that both pemoline and dextroamphetamine resulted in a significant reduction in symptoms as compared to placebo, with dextroamphetamine producing a more immediate and dramatic improvement and pemoline resulting in fewer side effects. *Millichap* (1973) and *Knights and Viets* (1973) reported the same results. Although research to date on this stimulant has been limited, the constant superiority over placebo, coupled with the absence of troublesome side effects, is very encouraging.

The effect of laevoamphetamine has been studied by *Arnold et al.* (1972) but will be discussed in the third part of this article.

We would also like to mention that the therapeutic effect of caffeine on hyperactive children has been investigated, but results are contradictory. *Schnackenberg* (1973) published the results of a pilot study in which 11 hyperactive children were treated with 200–300 mg of caffeine a day, in the form of one cup of coffee at breakfast, and a second cup at lunchtime. The teachers rating scale showed a marked improvement compared to the effect of previously administered Ritaline. *Firestone* (1974) confirmed this effect of caffeine. However, recent double-blind studies could not confirm the positive effect of caffeine on hyperactive children: *Garfinkel et al.* (1975) compared the effect of caffeine with the effect of methylfenidate and placebo in a double-blind cross-over study; 20 mg methylfenidate daily was significantly better than 160 mg caffeine in controlling behavior, especially impulsivity and hyperactivity. Only methylfenidate, but not caffeine was superior to decaffeinated coffee or placebo. We would like to remark that these researchers used a lower dosis of caffeine than *Schnackenberg.*

Lastly, we would like to mention a single trial of Captagon (Fenetyllin) 25–40 mg/day was given to hyperactive children; 16 of the 26 children showed a definite improvement, 6 improved slightly and 2 children deteriorated (*Mangold,* 1975). Further research, including double-blind cross-over studies are certainly necessary.

Nonstimulant Drugs

(A) Imipramine (Tofranil) is the tricyclic antidepressant which has had the most extensive trials in MBD. Several investigators have found imipramine to be effective in treating hyperactive children. *Huessy and Wright* (1970) and *Waizer et al.* (1974) treated hyperactive boys of elementary school age as outpatients with imipramine for 8 weeks, followed by 4 weeks of placebo. Ratings by a psychiatrist, parents and teachers indicated significant improvement in hyperactivity, attention span and sociability in the trial group. The usual dosis in *Waizer*'s study was 100–200 mg/day. This has been criticized by various researchers: *Saraf et al.* (1974) reported the sudden death of a 6-year-old girl after administration of an unusually large dosis of imipramine (14.7 mg/kg). *Winsberg et al.* (1974) noted the occurrence of seizures in seizure-free children following the administration of imipramine, and they also found electrocardiographic abnormalities. A total dose of 5 mg/kg of imipramine a day in three equal doses produced electrocardiographic changes in all of the 7 children (decreased amplitude and increased width of the T waves). We feel the safety margin of imipramine is too small, and that this drug should be used with precaution.

(B) *Major tranquillizers* such as chlorpromazine (Largactil), thiodorazine, melleril and haloperidol or haldol are often prescribed for hyperactive behavior. This is probably not recommended, as *Werry*'s (1970) study concluded that in natural settings, such as home and classroom, these drugs have no consistent effect on attention; the teachers evaluation was variable, with some reporting reduction in motor activity and others reporting decreased positive teacher-pupil interactions. On parent rating scales the children improved. In laboratory studies these drugs increased response latency and effected a deterioration in several kinds of task performance; *Werry* concluded that phenothiazines were generally inferior to stimulant drugs in effects on behavior and cognitive functioning. Side effects are also reported more frequently with phenothiazines.

(C) A pilot study undertaken by *David* on the effects of *lead chelation* therapy will be discussed later. This approach will probably become extremely important for selected MBD children.

(D) *Minor tranquillizers* are often prescribed for hyperkinetic behavior; but there does not seem to be sufficient evidence that these drugs are truly effective.

(E) *TRH* (thyreotropic releasing hormone) has been used by *Tiwary et al.* (1976), but only in 2 children. Behavior was significantly improved compared to a placebo injection, but this author has no explanation for this, and recommends further research.

(F) *Lithium* has also been used by several researchers, but when this drug is administered in a well-controlled trial, it does not seem to have any therapeutic effects on hyperkinetic behavior (*Whitehead and Clark,* 1970). Some authors feel that hyperkinetic behavior can be a masked hypomanic state in children, and suggest that lithium should be given prophylactically to children whose manic depressive parents responded favorably to lithium. Further research is obviously needed.

(G) *Antiepileptic drugs,* especially barbiturates, have a negative effect on hyperkinetic behavior (*Conners,* 1972).

(H) *Nootropic drugs,* such as Encephabol (Pyritinol hydrochloride) and Nootropil (Piracetam) are also without value in MBD.

Contribution of Pharmacological Research

MBD Children Can Be Divided in Several Subgroups, Depending on Their Response to Pharmacological Therapy

Most studies of MBD children selected on the basis of behavioral factors such as hyperactive motor behavior, decreased attention span, impulsiveness and a variety of cognitive and perceptual problems, show that these children can react in totally different ways to treatment with stimulant drugs. 40–70% improve, 5–20% show increased behavior problems. This variability in response to these drugs should stimulate further research into predictive criteria, and also indicates that there must be different subgroups amongst MBD patients, pathogenetically speaking. It is already known that children who react well to amphetamines, usually deteriorate when given barbiturates or major tranquillizers.

So far, research into predictive criteria of responders or nonresponders has not been able to show unanimous results (*Ross and Ross,* 1976). Criteria such as environmental, social and neurobiochemical factors, and neurological and EEG signs were investigated. Differentiation on an organic and nonorganic basis had no predictive value in several studies (*Werry and Sprague,* 1970; *Millichap and Boldrey,* 1967). Other researchers (*Buchsbaum and Wender,* 1973; *Satterfield et al.,* 1973) found that boys with minor neurological abnormalities such as equilibrium disorder, dysarthria, ambidextrity, and EEG abnormalities improved more than boys without these abnormalities. The degree of evidence of brain dysfunction correlated significantly with the probability of a good clinical response to stimulant drugs.

Sroufe (1975) remains fairly sceptical as to such correlations; he feels that no index of neurological status has yet been shown through cross-validation to have predictive utility and that physiological and psychological signs of drug response based on clinical experience are also empirically unsubstantiated.

Apart from a possible differentiation between positive and negative responders to stimulants, it should be born in mind that some MBD children respond well to one particular stimulant, but not to others. This means that in clinical practice one should be prepared to try several drugs if necessary (dexedrine, ritaline or pemoline).

Research by *Bradley* (1950), demonstrated that some children respond much better do *dl*-racemic amphetamine than to dextroamphetamine alone. This line of research prompted *Arnold et al.* (1972) to investigate the effectiveness of *d*- and *l*-amphetamine separately. This concerned a 9-week double-blind crossover comparison of dextroamphetamine, levoamphetamine and placebo; effects were assessed by a teacher rating scale, a parent rating scale, and a weekly quantification of parent-selected target symptoms.

Both active drugs were significantly more effective than placebo. Dextroamphetamine seemed consistently superior to levoamphetamine though not to a significant degree. Levoamphetamine seemed better for hyperactivity and aggressiveness than for inattentiveness, whereas dextroamphetamine seemed equally beneficial for all three factors. It was especially interesting that 2 children showed great improvement with levoamphetamine, but not at all with dextroamphetamine. These researchers then decided to test the hypothesis that the total MBD group contained a subgroup that could be described as 'unsocialized aggressive' (308.4) according to *Fish*'s (1971) criteria, and that this group of children might respond better to levoamphetamine than to dextroamphetamine. It is clinically very important to determine if there is a significant proportion of MBD children who might benefit more from levoamphetamine than from dexedrine. They explored this hypothesis in 1976 by selecting 31 children who complied with their criteria for MBD: children with such signs and symptoms as hyperactivity, distractability, short attention span, emotional lability, explosive behavior, incoordination, perceptual motor dysfunction and other minor neurological signs.

When the child was first seen, it was assigned to one of the three following diagnostic categories, described by *Fish* (1971):

308.0 hyperkinetic (immaturity, inadequacy, lability and poor organization).

308.2 overanxious (nervousness and possible hyperactivity with subjective distress, otherwise well organized).

308.4 unsocialized aggressive (aggressiveness and hostility with denial of feelings and personal responsibility, otherwise well organized).

These 31 children were studied in a double-blind crossover study of dextroamphetamine, levoamphetamine and placebo.

The 3 subgroups were compared on the following scales: (1) parent behavior checklist (Arnold and Smeltzer); (2) Conners' teachers rating scale; (3) David's hyperkinetic rating scale for parents; (4) David's hyperkinetic rating scale for teachers; (5) target symptom assessment (specific elements of the children's behavior considered as most troublesome by the parents).

In the unsocialized aggressive group, in contrast to the two other groups, 4 of the 5 scales show a trend for levoamphetamine to be slightly more effective than dextroamphetamine. It is important to note that 25 children reacted positively to medication; 14 children had better ratings on levoamphetamine (28%), and 4 children improved equally on either. These separate ratings were given at the end of the clinical study, before the code was broken by the physicians, who scored the total effect of the 3 drug conditions on a 9-point scale.

The authors conclude that there is a consistent trend that confirms their hypothesis that levoamphetamine is more effective than dextroamphetamine for the treatment of the unsocialized aggressive group, but they admit that they have not been able to prove it with statistically significant findings. They remain impressed by the clinical experience that levoamphetamine seems particularly effective for this particular group.

Dopamine Depletion

The fact that some MBD children show a spectacular improvement of their behavior when treated with stimulant drugs, and others with antidepressants suggests according to *Wender* (1974) that this type of drug treatment is in fact an intervention close to the origin of the causal chain in this syndrome. For the duration of their action, these drugs can produce immediate psychological growth. At such times these children may display more mature social, cognitive and interpersonal behavior than they have ever shown. As soon as the drug becomes inactive (e.g. 5th to 6th for dexedrine), the children revert to their former behavior. It is obviously not because a treatment is immediately beneficial to the patient that pathogenetical factors have been influenced, but it is certain that this type of behavior modification makes further hypotheses possible. Pharmacological research has demonstrated that amphetamine increases the amount of dopamine and norepinephrine at the synaptic clefts by a variety of mechanisms such as decreased neuronal uptake, increased granular release of catecholamines and decreased monoaminooxydase activity (*Snyder and Meyerhoff,* 1974).

A recent paper by *Schaywitz et al.* (1976b) seems to confirm the hypothesis that some MBD children in fact have a functional deficit in the dopaminergic synapses. The authors administered 6-hydroxydopamine to neonatal rats, and found a rapid and profound depletion of brain dopamine. The activity level of these rats, compared to that of normal rats, is comparable to the clinical hyperactivity seen in MBD children. During maturation, the activity of the rats with dopamine depletion decreased significantly when compared to controls. Once the rats attained sexual maturity (26th day), the activity levels in both groups was comparable. Brain dopamine concentrations in the 6-OHDA-treated rat pups were significantly lower than those found in their littermates, averaging 41.0% of controls of comparable age, while norepinephrine was reduced by only 8.3%. The authors also found that the 7 rats with a brain dopamine concentration of more than 55% of the mean concentration in the controls did not become hyperactive. On the other hand, the rats with much lower brain dopamine levels had extremely hyperkinetic behavior. These results clearly suggest that in rats, brain dopamine concentrations of less than 50–55% of untreated controls are a threshold for the production of hyperactivity.

Schaywitz et al. (1976a) published a sequel to this experiment. Dextroamphetamine or placebo was given to 6-OHDA-treated rats or to controls. When given dextroamphetamine, the controls showed increased activity, whereas the 6-OHDA-treated rats with dopamine depletion and hyperkinetc behavior showed a significant decrease in activity when compared to the placebo-treated rats.

Such findings suggest interesting further research, and will probably make an important contribution to the knowledge of the pathogenesis of the MBD syndrome.

Lead Chelation

The possibility that lead might be an etiological factor in hyperactivity was not investigated until recently. It was, however, already known that normal blood lead levels are at the most 40 μg%, and that clinical intoxication symptoms usually occur at levels above 80 μg% with encephalopathy and possible death at very high levels. Because lead encephalopathy can have hyperactivity as a possible sequel, and because blood levels between 40 and 80 μg% do not cause chemical lead intoxication, it seems reasonable to explore the effect of increased lead absorption on behavior.

David et al. (1972) published their first paper on the association of hyperactivity with increased body lead stores. Their findings indicated that children with no known cause of hyperactivity showed significantly raised lead levels as compared to the controls.

On the other hand, their patients with hyperactivity for which there was a highly probable etiology other than lead intoxication, showed no significant difference in lead values as compared to the controls. The lead levels found were above average, but lower than the toxic levels.

Silbergeld and Goldberg (1973) found support for a causal relationship between lead and a high degree of activity. Their first animal study in 1973 demonstrated that mice who had ingested lead from birth during 40–60 days, were more than three times as active as controls.

The fact that the doses of lead administered varied, and the fact that there were no deaths, suggests that hyperactivity may be a symptom occurring early in the period of exposure when the lead level is increased, but not toxic.

In their second study, *Silbergeld and Goldberg* (1974) replicated the causal relationship between lead ingestion and hyperactivity in mice, and then administered the stimulant drugs used in hyperactivity. Lead-treated mice responded with decreased hyperactivity to the stimulant medication, but with increased activity when given phenobarbital, as in humans. The controls showed opposite reactions. The parallels between this animal model of hyperactivity and clinical hyperactivity in children strongly suggested that lead might be an etiological agent in hyperactivity in children from urban areas.

David et al. (1976) published a pilot study, examining the effect of chelation on the behavioral problems of hyperkinetic children with elevated but nontoxic lead levels in blood and urine, i.e. greater than 25 μg/100 ml of blood and/or 80 μg/liter of urine. More than 50% of the hyperactive children referred to his study had elevated levels of lead in blood but levels lower than 60 μg%. The children with no known cause of hyperactivity showed a significant improvement when treated with chelating agents (Ca EDTA or penicillamine), when the teacher, parents or doctor rating scales were examined. Little or no improvement was seen in the behavior of the child with a probable cause for hyperactivity, other than an elevated lead level. This would seem to confirm that lead poisoning can have its clinical expression either as encephalopathy, if the lead levels are extreme, or as hyperactive behavior, if lower lead levels are present.

This therapy with chelating agents is a possibility, only if no other causes for the behavioral problem are found, and if a moderate increase in blood lead values exists.

Practical Conclusions for Clinical Use of Drugs in the MBD Syndrome

Drug therapy is only one of the multiple types of possible therapy for MBD children; other methods include remedial education, residential treatment, special education programs such as a minimal stimulation program, individual and group psychotherapy of MBD children, group therapy with parents (*Feighner and Feighner,* 1974), individual parent counselling behavior therapy at home or in the classroom, music therapy, etc.

Some professionals, such as *Cruickshank et al.* (1961) with their minimal stimulation program, refuse to treat children undergoing drug therapy. Others feel that the only possible approach is pharmacological; *Friedman et al.* (1973) for example, concluded that an 8-month trial of stimulants alone, or a combined therapy with stimulant drugs and educational group therapy and parent-group counselling, had identical results.

Drug therapy certainly has a place in MBD therapy, but we feel that the following two basic questions should be answered beforehand: (1) At what level is therapy indicated? That is, should we try to treat the causes, the pathogenetical mechanisms, the syndrome or the symptoms? (2) How do the possible therapeutic gains compare to the eventual side effects? Long-term as well as short-term side effects should be examined.

Clinical practice should also take the following factors in account, namely (1) the realistic possibilities of the proposed therapy which are determined by geographical factors, motivation and the availability of well-trained and efficient therapists, and (2) the amount of time and energy that the therapists will have to invest, and the final cost of the chosen therapy for the family and for society in general.

Level of Therapy

(A) If the primary cause is still operational, then it must obviously be treated first. Lead chelation therapy will probably be one of the possible causal approaches, but further studies and confirmation of *David*'s conclusions are essential. Another example of a primary cause is an unstructured family setting or school environment, and it will be essential to try to change this (*Kok,* 1978).

(B) In most MBD children, however, no immediate causal factor can be found, but the etiology could be genetic (*Wender,* 1974), or a sequel to brain damage. If distractibility and hyperkinetic behavior is a central problem in these children, a functional deficit in brain dopamine and norepinephrine in certain synapses can be postulated. This functional deficit can be corrected by administering stimulant drugs, which are known to increase brain dopamine. This type of therapy we would consider as effecting the pathogenetical mechanisms.

As long as predictive criteria have not been clearly defined, this type of therapy will be dependent on a clinical trial for each child. If a spectacular improvement in behavior occurs, it will confirm the diagnosis of this particular type of MBD. Further pharmacological and clinical research will probably be able to differentiate several subtypes of MBD syndromes, based for example on biochemical factors. This means that in our opinion, stimulant drug therapy is not the first choice for the whole group of MBD children, and should only be used when hyperactivity and distractability are the main problems.

On the other hand, stimulant drug therapy should be extended to children with hyperactivity and distractability without minimal brain dysfunction, but with global brain dysfunction, as mentally handicapped children or epileptics, in whom antiepileptic drugs very often worsen such symptoms as distractability and hyperkinetic behavior. This point of view is held by several researchers, and is confirmed by our own experience.

It is not always the case that stimulant drug therapy improves behavior to such an extent that counselling of parents and teachers need be kept to a minimum. Most children show a moderate improvement without presenting normal behavior, and intensive counselling of parents and teachers will then be necessary during the whole period of treatment.

(C) If causal therapy is impossible and if the pathogenetical mechanisms cannot be influenced, syndromatic or symptomatic treatment is indicated.

Syndromatic treatment would be a minimal stimulation environment, behavior modification techniques at home and at school, and counselling of the parents as to how to modify the home environment. A referral to a special school or to a residential treatment center can be necessary. An example of syndromal therapy is the 'Minimal Stimulation Program' developed by *Cruickshank et al.* (1961). *Kok* (1972) was the first to work out a residential therapy for children he calls 'structopathic' children.

Finally, it can be necessary to treat certain children with too disturbing behavioral variations with drugs, such as major tranquillizers; this type of approach we would call symptomatic therapy. Other therapeutic approaches can be necessary for symptoms such as perceptual disorders, which can be improved with remedial training. Secondary effects of the MBD syndrome such as neurotic behavior or scapegoating by the family must be recognized and treated, either by individual therapy or family therapy.

Possible Disadvantages of Drug Therapy

The second problem in MBD therapy is the evaluation of the disadvantages, which should certainly not outweigh the therapeutic benefits. We would first of all like to point out that far more extensive studies are necessary on larger populations and with a much larger follow-up. As far as we know, the short-term side effects are temporary, and are less pronounced when using Pemoline or Ritalin than amphetamines, which is why we personally prefer these two drugs. The long-term side effects are less well known, but there has been no evidence so far that these stimulant drugs can lead to addiction, if these drugs are limited to the 6- to 12-year-old children (*Beck et al.*, 1975). Some investigators even feel that stimulant drugs can be continued during puberty and adolescence, if the MBD syndrome persists. We do not have any personal experience with this problem, but we do feel that stimulant drugs should be used with great caution after the age of 14. As to the effect of these drugs on growth, there seems to be sufficient evidence that a catch-up occurs after drug termination. In any case, stimulant drugs should not be given during the summer holidays. With these simple precautions, there seems to be no danger of growth retardation. We do feel, however, that the prescribing of stimulant drugs should be a responsible medical decision, and should not be taken because of parental pressure, without a thorough evaluation of the child himself. Inability of teachers or parents to cope with normal active children is not an indication for drug therapy.

References

Arnold, L.; Wender, P.H.; McCloskey, K., and Snyder, S.H.: Levoamphetamine and dextroamphetamine. Comparative efficacy in the hyperkinetic syndrome. Archs gen. Psychiat. *27:* 816–822 (1972).

Beck, L.; Langford, W.; Mackey, M., and Sum, C.: Childhood chemotherapy and later drug abuse and growth curve. A follow-up study of 30 adolescents. Am. J. Psychiat. *132:* 436–438 (1975).

Bradley, C.: Benzedrine and dexedrine in the treatment of children's behaviour disorders. Pediatrics, Springfield *5:* 24–37 (1950).

Buchsbaum, M. and Wender, P.: Average evoked responses in normal and minimally brain dysfunctioned children treated with amphetamine. Preliminary report. Archs gen. Psychiat. *29:* 764–770 (1973).

Cantwell, D.: A model for investigation of psychiatric disorders in childhood; in *Anthony* Explorations in child psychiatry, pp. 57–80 (Holt, Reineman Winston, London/New York 1975).

Conners, C.K.: Recent drug studies with hyperkinetic children. J. Learn. Disabil. *4:* 476–483 (1971).

Conners, C.K.: Pharmacotherapy of psychopathology in children; in *Quay and Werry* Psychopathological disorders of childhood, pp. 316–347 (Wiley, New York 1972).

Conners, C.K.; Taylor, E.; Meo, G.; Kurtz, M.A., and Fournier, M.: Magnesium pemoline and dextroamphetamine. A controlled study in children with minimal brain dysfunction. Psychopharmacologia *26:* 321–336 (1972).

Cruickshank, W.M.; Bentzen, F.A.; Ratzeburg, F.H., and Tannhauser, M.T.: A teaching method for brain injured and hyperactive children (Syracuse University Press, Syracuse 1961).

David, O.J.; Clark, J., and Voeller, K.: Lead and hyperactivity. Lancet *ii:* 900–903 (1972).

David, O.J.; Hoffmann, S.P.; Sverd, J.; Clark, J., and Voeller, K.: Lead and hyperactivity. Behavioural response to cholation. A pilot study. Am. J. Psychiat. *133:* 1155–1158 (1976).

Denckla, M.B.; Bemporad, J.R., and MacKey, M.L.: Tics following methylfenidate administration. J. Am. med. Ass. *235:* 1349–1351 (1976).

Ellis, M.J.; Witt, P.A.; Reynolds, R., and Sprague, R.L.: Methylphenidate and the activity of hyperactives in the informal setting. Child Dev. *45:* 217–220 (1974).

Feighner, A.C. and Feighner, J.P.: Multimodality treatment of the hyperkinetic child. Am. J. Psychiat. *131:* 459–463 (1974).

Firestone, P.: The effects of reinforcement contingencies and caffeine on hyperactive children; Diss. Montreal (unpubl. 1974).

Fish, B.: The 'one child, one drug' myth of stimulants in hyperkinesis. Importance of diagnostic categories in evaluating treatment. Archs gen. Psychiat. *25:* 193–203 (1971).

Friedman, R.; Dale, E.P., and Wagner, J.H.: A long-term comparison of two treatment regimens for minimal brain dysfunction. Drug therapy versus combined therapy. Clin. Pediatr. *12:* 666–671 (1973).

Garfinkel, B.D.; Webster, C.D., and Sloman, L.: Methylphenidate and caffeine in the treatment of children with minimal brain dysfunction. Am. J. Psychiat. *132:* 723–728 (1975).

Huessy, H.R. and Wright, A.L.: The use of imipramine in children's behavior disorders. Acta paedopsychiat. *37:* 194–199 (1970).

Knights, R.M. and Viets, C.A.: The effects of pemoline on hyperactive boys (Department of Psychology, Carleton University, Ottawa 1973).

Kok, J.F.W.: Structopathic children. Results of experimental research of structuring group therapy (Rotterdam University Press, Rotterdam 1972).

Kok, J.F.M.: Structuurzwakte door opvoeding. Tijdschr. Orthoped. Kinderpsych. *3:* 14–22 (1978).

Mangold, B.: Medikamentöse Behandlung des Minimal Brain Dysfunction Syndrom. Prax. Kinderpsychol. Kinderpsychiatrie, pp. 185–190 (1976).

Millichap, J.G.: Drugs in management of minimal brain dysfunction. Ann. N.Y. Acad. Sci. *205:* 321–334 (1973).

Millichap, J.G. and Boldrey, E.S.: Studies in hyperkinetic behaviour. II. Laboratory and clinical evolutions of drug treatments. Neurology, Minneap. *17:* 467–471, 519 (1967).

Pyck, K.: The use of drugs in the treatment of hyperkinetic children. A pilot study. 2nd Int. Congr. on Learning Disabilities, Brussels 1975 (unpubl.)

Ross, D.M. and Ross, S.A.: Hyperactivity. Research, theory, and action (Wiley, New York 1976).

Safer, D.J. and Allen, R.P.: Hyperactive children, diagnosis and management (University Park Press, Baltimore 1976).

Saraf, K.R.; Klein, D.F.; Gittelman-Klein, R., and Groff, S.: Imipramine side effects in children. Psychopharmacologia *37:* 265–274 (1974).

Satterfield, J.H.; Cantwell, D.P.; Saul, R.E.; Lesser, L.I., and Podosin, R.L.: Response to stimulant drug treatment in hyperactive children, prediction from E.E.G. and neurological findings. J. Autism Childh. Schiz. *3:* 36–48 (1973).

Schaywitz, B.A.; Klopper, J.H.; Yager, R.D., and Gordon, J.W.: Paradoxical response to amphetamine in developing rats treated with 6-hydroxydopamine. Nature, Lond. *261:* 153–155 (1976a).

Schaywitz, B.A.; Yager, R.D., and Klopper, J.H.: Selective brain dopamine depletion in developing rats. An experimental model of minimal brain dysfunction. Science *191:* 305–308 (1976b).

Schnackenberg, R.C.: Caffeine as a substitute for Schedule II stimulants in hyperkinetic children. Am. J. Psychiat. *130:* 796–798 (1973).

Silbergeld, E.K. and Goldberg, A.M.: A lead-induced behavioral disorder. Life Sci. *13:* 1275–1283 (1973).

Silbergeld, E.K. and Goldberg, A.M.: Lead-induced behavioral dysfunction. An animal model of hyperactivity. Expl Neurol. *42:* 146–157 (1974).

Snyder, S.M. and Meyerhoff, J.L.: Ann. N.Y. Acad. Sci. *14:* 1605–1621 (1974).

Sprague, R.L.; Barnes, K.R., and Werry, J.S.: Methylphenidate and thioridazine. Learning, activity, and behavior in emotionally disturbed boys. Am. J. Orthopsychiat. *40:* 615–628 (1970).

Sroufe, L.A.: Drug treatment of children with behavior problems; in *Horowitz* Review of child development research, vol. 4 (University of Chicago Press, Chicago 1975).

Sykes, D.H.; Douglas, V.I., and Morgenstern, G.: The effect of methylphenidate (Ritalin) on sustained attention in hyperactive children. Psychopharmacologia *25:* 262–274 (1972).

Tiwary, C.M.; Rosenbloom, A.L.; Robertson, M.F., and Parker, J.C.: Effects of thyreotropin-releasing hormone in minimal brain dysfunction. Pediatrics, Springfield *56:* 119–121 (1975).

Waizer, J.; Hoffman, S.P.; Polizos, P., and Engelhardt, D.M.: Outpatient treatment of hyperactive school children with imipramine. Am. J. Psychiat. *131:* 587–591 (1974).

Wender, P.H.: Minimal brain dysfunction in children (Wiley-Interscience, New York 1971).

Wender, P.H.: Some speculations concerning a possible biochemical basis of minimal brain dysfunction. Life Sci. *14:* 1605–1621 (1974).

Werry, J.S.: Some clinical and laboratory studies of psychotropic drugs in children. An overview; in *Smith* Drugs and cerebral function (Thomas, Springfield 1970).

Werry, J.S. and Sprague, R.L.: Hyperactivity; in *Costello* Symptoms of psychopathology, pp. 397–417 (Wiley, New York 1970).

Whitehead, P.L. and Clark, L.D.: Effect of lithium carbonate, placebo, and thioridazine on hyperactive children. Am. J. Psychiat. *127:* 824–825 (1970).

Winsberg, B.G.; Goldstein, S.; Yepes, L.E., and Perel, J.M.: Imipramine electrocardiographic abnormalities in hyperactive children. Am. J. Psychiat. *132:* 542–545 (1975).

K. Pyck, MD, Reader in Child Psychiatry and *P. Baines,* MD, Pediatrician, Assistant in Child Psychiatry, University of Leuven, Child Psychiatry Unit, University Hospital, Gasthuisberg, *Leuven* (Belgium)

Adv. biol. Psychiat., vol. 1, pp. 84–95 (Karger, Basel 1978)

Animal Hyperactivity Syndromes: Do they have any Relevance to Minimal Brain Dysfunction

D.G. Grahame-Smith

MRC Unit and University Department of Clinical Pharmacology, Radcliffe Infirmary, Oxford

Extrapolation from observations of animal behaviour to human behaviour and mental processes is always fraught with difficulty. It is difficult enough when considering generally accepted and fairly well defined psychiatric syndromes such as manic-depressive disease and schizophrenia, but the position is even more difficult when considering the syndrome in childhood called 'minimal brain dysfunction'. The number of different titles the syndrome has received, e.g. minimal brain dysfunction, minimal cerebral dysfunction, the hyperkinetic syndrome, and the hyperactive child; specific learning disabilities (*Wender,* 1975) show its complexity and variability. Some of course, doubt whether the syndrome exists in neurologically normal children, and believe that this 'syndrome' of behavioural disorders is just one way that 'normal' children behave. Obviously to make any headway in relating animal behaviour to the clinical syndrome of minimal brain dysfunction, I am put in the position of having to accept, for the sake of the discussion, that the syndrome does exist. One thing I am prepared to accept is that there are certain behavioural disorders in children covered by the term minimal brain dysfunction, which in the eyes of observers (child psychiatrists, parents and teachers) do seem to 'improve', at least in the short term, when these children are given *d*-amphetamine or methylphenidate. This does not mean, of course, that the behaviour is abnormal, for there are all sorts of normal behaviour and emotions which can be manipulated with drugs which alter the mind. Conviviality at social occasions is frequently improved by alcohol but that does not mean that lack of conviviality on such occasions is abnormal.

Hyperactivity rarely presents as an isolated symptom (*Millichap,* 1976). Often, it is associated with a short attention span, distractibility, impulsiveness, inco-ordination, perceptual impairment and disorders of memory and learning. Indeed hyperactivity (depending on definition) may occur in only 75% of patients and some children with other features of the symptom complex may be placid and inert and 20% have normal patterns of activity. Therefore, the simple examination of hyperactivity in animals is only likely to shed light on one particular symptom of the clinical condition and at the outset it is apparent that other behavioural disorders in animals may tell us, as much or more than mere observation of locomotor activity.

What is one looking for in animals which might bear relevance to the minimal brain dysfunction syndrome? The affected children are excessively active, always on the go, running rather than walking, always into things. At school the child will not sit still at his desk, frequently gets up from his seat, walks around the room, humming, whistling and tapping and generally bothers people (*Wender,* 1975). General overall activity may not be much increased but there does seem to be an inappropriateness to it. This inappropriate hyperactivity seems to diminish at puberty. Disturbances of fine co-ordination are prominent in these children, something which is not usually analysed in animal hyperactivity syndromes. Although some features of the minimal brain dysfunction syndrome, such as attentional difficulties, impulsivity, problems with social relationships and memory and learning are to some extent amenable to analysis in animals, not much work has been done on these features in the animal hyperactivity syndromes of relevance to the minimal brain dysfunction syndrome.

Now, when one speaks of hyperactivity syndromes in animals one is speaking really of rats, in which, for the sake of expediency and cost most studies have been done. So, one immediately sees a problem. What on earth is one likely to learn about a complex behavioural disorder such as the MBD syndrome by watching and measuring the locomotor activity of a rat in a cage? Obviously little. The strategy though is to produce disturbances in locomotor activity and other behavioural sets by pharmacological means and brain lesions of one sort or another and consider how these might relate to the MBD syndrome. In this one is constantly brought back to the effects of amphetamine and methylphenidate. Other drugs such as the tricyclic antidepressants have been used with some success in the MBD syndrome but amphetamines and methylphenidate have the most striking effects. The clinical actions of these drugs are important. The children become calmer, their attentional span increases, their social behaviour becomes more acceptable, they become socially more responsive and aware of their effects on others. They improve in their ability to think ahead and surprisingly the control of their hyperactivity may be accompanied by improvement in fine co-ordination. There is some controversy whether all this, in the long term, results in an improvement on learning.

It is frequently thought that these effects of amphetamine and methylphenidate in children with the MBD syndrome are paradoxical when compared with the effects of these drugs in adults. This point will be examined in detail later because it is an important one but suffice it to say here that children treated with amphetamines may display anorexia, insomnia and signs of arousal if the dose of amphetamine is too high, features which adults show. The paradox lies in the apparent calming of the hyperactive child as compared with the alerting, exciting and euphoriant effects of amphetamines in 'normal' adults. This paradox may only be a superficial one and can I believe, be explained.

Hyperactivity Syndromes in the Rat

What is 'a hyperactivity syndrome', in the rat? The first consideration is, of course, the mode of activity the level of which one wishes to observe. 'Hyperactivity' is a blanket term and needs definition. Most of the hyperactive syndromes involve one or the other of two behavioural modes, i.e., locomotor activity (walking or running about) and/or repetitive types of behaviour (stereotypes). Locomotor activity can be observed by the breakage of photocell beams, tipping of cages breaking contacts, or on activity meters such as the Animex activity meter which I and my colleagues use. All of these methods measure certain types of locomotor acitivty and observation of the rat is important so that the quality of behaviour can be determined. Movement in tunnels or mazes, on hole-boards, in open fields, etc., measure other sorts of locomotor activity perhaps associated with exploratory activity. One is forced to confess that, particularly with increased locomotor activity produced by drugs, the quality and behavioural meaning of the increase has not been carefully analysed, since the increased locomotor activity is often only being used as an index of the degree of drug action, rather than being studied in its own right. Much more needs to be known about the meaning of increased locomotor activity in response to drugs and brain lesions.

Stereotyped behaviours consist of repetitive actions, seemingly meaningless in the context of integrated behaviour, and consist of repetitive grooming, sniffing, head weaving, gnawing, licking, rearing or forepaw padding depending upon the pharmacological challenge. Most of the pharmacological treatments which produce increased locomotor activity also produce stereotyped behaviour patterns and this important consideration will be discussed later.

In table I are shown a number of hyperactivity syndromes in rats produced by various manoeuvres.

'Dopaminergic' Hyperactivity Syndromes

Much the same syndrome can be produced by *L*-dopa plus a MAO inhibitor, amphetamine, methylphenidate or apomorphine with differences in the time course of behavioural events, intensity and duration but with qualitatively similar features.

L-Dopa and a MAO inhibitor are thought to increase dopaminergic stimulation in the brain by increasing dopamine synthesis with consequent 'spill-over' of

Table I. Hyperactivity syndromes in the rat

1 'Dopaminergic'
L-Dopa + MAO inhibitor
Amphetamine
Methylphenidate
Apomorphine
2 'Serotonergic'
Tryptophan or 5-hydroxytryptophan
+ a MAO inhibitor
5-Methoxy-N,N′-dimethyltryptamine (+ other tryptamine derivatives)
3 Serotonin depletion (?)
p-Chlorophenylalanine
Median raphé nuclei lesions
4 Chronic neuroleptic administration (α-flupenthixol)
5 Hyperactivity and lead
6 Ventral tegmental area syndrome
Social deprivation – isolation

dopamine from nerve endings onto post-synaptic dopamine receptors with a resulting increase in the functional activity of dopamine.

Amphetamine is thought to produce its effects by releasing dopamine from dopaminergic nerve endings onto post-synaptic receptor sites.

Methylphenidate is generally thought to act in much the same way as amphetamine though pharmacological differences can be discerned (*Thornburg and Moore,* 1973). Both amphetamine and methylphenidate also block dopamine reuptake. Apomorphine is thought to act as a direct dopamine agonist.

This dopaminergic syndrome in its least intense form is characterised by apparently aimless increased locomotor activity. Superficially, it might be suspected that increased exploration is the reason. However, as *Randrup and Munkrad* (1974) have beautifully shown, there is often a stereotyped quality to this increased locomotor activity reminiscient of soldiers with mine detectors scanning a minefield! With larger doses of these drugs or later on in the syndrome with a particular dose stereotyped behavioural modes set in. Sniffing, rearing, licking, gnawing and spurts of backward locomotion occur. So great may this stereotyped behaviour become that 'hyperactivity', in the sense of increased ambulatory locomotor activity, ceases and there is plainly a gross restriction of the number of types of behaviour the rat is capable of. To my mind this gross stereotyped behaviour is evidence of behavioural drug 'toxicity'. This is not to say that consideration of it cannot be heuristically useful.

Treatments such as these probably have a global effect to increase dopaminergic function in the brain and so the question arises as to whether all the features of the 'dopaminergic hyperactivity syndrome', i.e. locomotor activity and stereotyped behaviour, are mediated by the same neuronal pathways.

Using different techniques *Iversen and Kelly* (1975) and *Jackson et al.* (1975) have reached similar conclusions. Functional dopamine activity in the mesolimbic system served by the nucleus accumbens is necessary for dopaminergic mediated locomotor activity while functional dopaminergic activity in the nigrostriatal system is necessary for stereotyped behaviour. These experiments provide an important precedent. That is, that although pharmacological treatments may have a specific pharmacological action (e.g. dopaminergic stimulation), such an action may occur at many different sites in the brain. This results in a complex behavioural pattern analysis of which reveals that the various components are dependent upon the functioning of different neuronal tracts.

It also seems that different forms of behaviour have different pharmacological sensitivities, e.g. low doses of amphetamines produce only increased locomotor activity, higher doses produce initially locomotor activity passing into stereotyped behaviour. Perhaps this indicates neural substrates with differing sensitivities to amphetamine though I must confess I find it difficult to understand this temporal development of complex behavioural patterns in response to centrally active drugs.

'Serotonergic' Hyperactivity Syndrome

Hess and Doepfner (1961) first described a behavioural syndrome of which hyperactivity is a part, resulting from the administration of *L*-tryptophan and a MAO inhibitor to rats. The biochemical and pharmacological basis of this syndrome and its dependence upon brain 5-hydroxytryptamine was later studied in detail (*Grahame-Smith,* 1971) and the matter has been reviewed recently (*Green and Grahame-Smith,* 1976).

The syndrome can be produced by *L*-tryptophan or *L*-5-hydroxytryptophan plus a MAO inhibitor. These treatments increase brain 5-hydroxytryptamine (5-HT) concentrations very greatly and it is presumed 5-HT 'spills over' from 5-HT nerve endings onto post-synaptic 5-HT receptors. A similar syndrome, but with a different time course can be produced by 5-methoxy-N,N-dimethyl-tryptamine which is presumed to act as a direct 5-HT agonist, as are several other tryptamine derivatives.

In some ways the syndrome is not unlike the 'dopaminergic hyperactivity' syndrome with increased locomotor activity plus stereotyped behaviours. The locomotor activity increase is indistinguishable in its early phase though later on in the syndrome the hind legs become abducted and the belly is nearer the floor of the cage. The stereotyped behaviour does differ though. During the increased locomotor activity the rats are hyperactive to handling (though not aggressive as they may be in the dopaminergic syndrome), they squeak when bumped against by another rat. Then as the syndrome progresses a fine body tremor can be seen and felt, the rat becomes rigid when picked up, the hindlegs are abducted, lateral head weaving, alternate forepaw padding and hyperpyrexia occur. If the dose of the treatment is high opisthotonus, chronic fits and death ensue. The head weaving and alternate forepaw padding are striking stereotyped behaviours, which in their intensity, I believe distinguish this syndrome from the 'dopaminergic' syndrome.

There is little doubt on the biochemical and pharmacological front that this syndrome is due to 5-HT, though there does seem to be an important permissive or 'linking' role for dopaminergic mechanisms in the behavioural expression of certain features of the syndrome (*Green and Grahame-Smith,* 1974).

Jacobs et al. (1977) have performed various brain lesions in an attempt to define broadly those neural pathways responsible for the syndrome. Surprisingly (to me), they have found that the stereotyped behaviour persists even when the neuraxis is completely transected at the caudal mesencephalic level, posterior to the red nucleus, substantia nigra and dorsal and median raphé nuclei. It appears, therefore, that lower brain stem and spinal cord are sufficient for certain of the stereotypic behavioural features. Full anatomical analysis of all the features of the syndrome is yet awaited.

'Serotonin Depletion' Hyperactivity

There is some controversy here between *Jacobs et al.* (1977) and *Hole et al.* (1976). *Jacobs et al.* (1977) found that *p*-chlorophenylalanine, which inhibits tryptophan 5-hydroxylase and blocks the synthesis of brain 5-HT and lowers its brain concentration, causes increased locomotor activity. *Jacobs* also found that lesions of the median raphé nuclei caused increased locomotor activity and potentiated the locomotor response to amphetamine. He went on to show that median raphé nuclei lesions depleted hippocampal 5-HT and that removal of the hippocampus blocked the hyperactivity produced by both median raphé nuclei lesions and *p*-chlorophenylalanine.

Jacobs and Cohen (1975) also showed that in rats with median raphé nuclei lesions the type of increased behavioural activity was characteristic, with darting from corner to corner of the cage. Different types of behaviour were found to be abnormal with dorsal raphé nuclei lesions. The raphé nuclei 'house' most of the serotonergic nerve cell bodies in the brain. It seems very likely that different subsets of serotonergic neurons subserve different types of behaviour.

Hole et al. (1976) have, however, been unable to replicate *Jacobs'* results by neurotoxic lesions of the medical 5-HT bundle with 5,7-dihydroxytryptamine. They found their lesions reduced activity and they have raised the question whether *Jacobs'* lesions were interfering with the function of some other neurotransmitter pathway.

Social Deprivation

Valzelli (1973) described increased spontaneous locomotor activity and exaggerated responses to the environment in mice which had been isolated.

Sahakian et al. (1975) showed that this also occurred in rats reared in isolation. These rats show increased spontaneous locomotor activity and an increased sensitivity of stereotyped behaviour but not locomotor activity to amphetamine.

Chronic Neuroleptic Administration (α-Flupenthixol)

For some time it has been known that when rats are given neuroleptic drugs (certain phenothiazines, thioxanthenes and butyrophenones) chronically, then subsequently the locomotor response to treatments increasing dopaminergic activity in the brain is increased (*Heal et al.*, 1976). *Heal et al.* (1976) also showed that of chlorpromazine, α-flupenthixol, spiroperidol and haloperidol, only chlorpromazine enhanced the hyperactivity syndrome produced by increasing serotonergic activity in the brain, the others producing enhanced responses only to increases in dopaminergic activity.

The current view of the mode of the acute action of neuroleptic drugs is that they block the action of dopamine to stimulate dopamine-sensitive adenylate cyclase in certain areas of the brain (*Iversen*, 1975). This can be shown *in vitro* and recently this has also been shown *in vivo* (*Heal et al.*, unpubl. observations, 1977). However, when these drugs are given chronically and with the correct experimental protocol clear enhancement of dopaminergic behavioural activity can be elicited. It has been suggested quite reasonably that this indicates receptor supersensitivity to dopamine induced by chronic dopamine blockade but we have so far been unable to find evidence for this by studying dopamine sensitive adenylate cyclase.

Whatever the mechanism though, behavioural supersensitivity to 5-HT and dopamine can be induced by appropriate neuroleptics given by appropriate schedules.

Sahakian et al. (1976) gave α-flupenthixol chronically to rats (a fairly specific dopamine antagonist) and found that spontaneous locomotor activity was increased and that sniffing stereotyped behaviour also sometimes occurred. Other aspects of behaviour have not, as far as I know, been studied in detail.

One would suspect that this increased spontaneous activity seen after chronic neuroleptic administration is also related to increased brain dopaminergic activity, though that would be speculative at present. All the indications are that the response to amphetamine in these animals would be an enhancement of amphetamine's effects, i.e. a greatly increased response in terms of locomotor activity, rather than a diminution.

Hyperactivity and Lead

Sauerhoff and Michaelson (1973) reported that newborn rats suckling mothers eating a diet containing 4% lead carbonate displayed increased locomotor activity, aggressiveness and excessive stereotyped behaviour (e.g., self-grooming) starting at 4 weeks of age. This syndrome was accompanied by a 20% decrease in whole brain dopamine concentrations. As far as I am aware the effect of amphetamine on this syndrome has not been studied, the regional distribution of the dopamine loss has not been looked at, nor has the behavioural disturbance really been analysed in detail. It would be worthwhile looking at these factors to see if there is any link here with the ventral tegmental syndrome (see below).

The Ventral Tegmental Syndrome

Le Moal and his colleagues in 1969 described a very interesting behavioural syndrome in rats resulting from radio frequency (RF) lesions of the ventral mesencephalic tegmentum (VMT). This behavioural syndrome is reviewed by *Le Moal et al.* (1977) and the details of its neuroanatomy, neuropharmacology and neurobiochemistry by *Tassin et al.* (1977).

The behavioural syndrome described is a complex one. It consists of increased locomotor activity (2–3 times appropriate controls), no change in sleep time, difficulties in suppressing previous learned responses, difficulty in tolerating frustrating situations, inability to learn a passive avoidance test, in addition to other features. *Le Moal* and his colleagues bring out an important feature of the locomotor activity. In an open field situation or in the hole-board exploratory test, although there is increased locomotor activity in the lesioned animals, it does not seem to indicate increased exploratory activity. Another very interesting feature is the effect of the lesion on food handling. In a free situation the cage of these animals becomes messy with food crumbs. When placed in an open field with access to a home cage, many of the lesioned animals as compared with appropriate controls no longer hoard food, eating in the open field rather than taking the food back to the home cage to eat it. The lesioned rats are disturbed by anything in their environment and do not interpret environmental cues appropriately. *Le Moal et al.* (1977) state: 'Though fundamental behaviours were not quantitatively impaired they seemed qualitatively disorganised' and conlude 'The lesioned rats are underaroused and are not able to respond accurately to the environment, where cues are not integrated or to compete for food or anything, or to produce organised behaviour for security.'

The lesion in the VMT area is in the area of the A10 group of dopaminergic neuronal cell bodies. The behavioural syndrome can be produced by lesions in this area brought about either by radio frequency or by 6-hydroxydopamine microinjections into the area. These lesions produced a marked fall in the dopamine content of the orbito-frontal cortex and accumbens and this fall correlates very well with the increase in locomotor activity. The ventral tegmental area also contains numerous ascending serotonergic fibres and marked changes of 5-HT levels were found in the cerebral cortex of lesioned rats. However, no significant correlation could be found between the fall in cerebral cortical 5-HT and increased activity. Similar lack of correlations was found for striatal dopamine and noradrenaline in the frontal cortex.

When lesioned animals were treated chronically with *d*-amphetamine (1–2 mg/kg) there was no effect on the locomotor activity of normal animals, whereas in those animals with RF-VMT lesions the hyperactivity which normally appeared was progressively reduced to that of normal rats. Acute apomorphine administration also reduced activity in lesioned animals to normal levels.

Le Moal et al. (1977) propose that the VMT-A10 area syndrome may be similar to the minimal brain dysfunction syndrome, that the behavioural disturbance in the lesioned rats can be linked to the disturbance in the affected children's behaviour and that the response to amphetamine in the lesioned rats can be extrapolated to the MBD syndrome. One point which cannot be easily explained at the moment is the action of amphetamine. If the VMT-A10 lesion destroys dopaminergic mesocortical neurones, then it is unlikely that amphetamine is acting by releasing dopamine from dead dopaminergic neurones in the cortex. Of course amphetamine may be releasing dopamine from cortical nerve endings which have not been destroyed thus increasing cortical dopaminergic activity or acting through some other mechanism.

Conclusions

Where then do all these studies take us in regard to the minimal brain dysfunction syndrome? Consistently, one is brought back to the effects of amphetamine and methylphenidate as clues to some disturbance of brain function in these children.

Sahakian and Robbins (1977) have been drawn to the conclusion that the action of amphetamine in MBD to decrease activity and improve attention and concentration is tied up with its ability to produce stereotyped behaviour. Amphetamine can produce stereotyped behaviour patterns in adults (*Rylander,* 1971) and the behaviour becomes increasingly perseversative and 'constricted' with increasing dosage of the drug. In rats simple locomotor activity produced by low doses of amphetamine disappears as stereotyped behaviour becomes prominent with larger doses. As already pointed out these two types of behaviour can be neuroanatomically and behaviourally separated.

Sahakian and Robbins (1977) point out that stereotyped behaviour appears as a restriction of the number of items of behaviour the animal will perform.

Along with *Sroufe and Steward* (1973), they interpret the action of amphetamine and methylphenidate in the following way (at least this is my interpretation of their hypothesis). Children with MBD have a dysfunction of the brain which interferes with attention. These children then lack concentration and are easily distracted and impulsive and perhaps the increased activity they show is secondary to this. What amphetamine and methylphenidate then do is to produce some stereotypy of behaviour so that behaviour becomes constricted and the child performs the task presented to it (i.e. because amphetamine stereotypes behaviour in animals and man, it concentrates the mind to the task in hand). *Sroufe and Steward* (1973) argue that amphetamine and methylphenidate produce behaviour in children with MBD so that 'performance is improved on repetitive, routinised tasks that require sustained attention'.

This hypothesis concerning the extrapolation of the behavioural effects of amphetamine and methylphenidate in animals to their effects in children with the MBD syndrome in fact fits in very nicely with the effects of amphetamine in the ventral tegmental syndrome previously described. If the ventral tegmental syndrome is considered as a disorganisation of behaviour produced by a depletion of cortical dopamine, resulting in easy distractibility, lack of proper interpretation of environmental cues, non-exploratory increased locomotor activity and lack of organised behaviour for security, then the effect of amphetamine (and apomorphine) to increase dopaminergic activity in the brain and to produce behaviourally a tendency toward stereotype of behaviour 'allows' the animal to 'concentrate' on the task in hand, organise its behaviour and results in a decrease in its aimless and pointless hyperactivity.

I find the hypothesis of *Sahakian and Robbins* (1975) on the behavioural actions of amphetamine linked with the findings of *Le Moal* and *Tassin* on the ventral tegmental syndrome really rather compelling as a model upon which to think about the biology of minimal brain dysfunction.

The other hyperactivity syndromes are important in understanding the modes of behaviour which can be produced by manipulating brain monoamine function and they provide an experimental background for understanding the pharmacological and behavioural actions of amphetamine and methylphenidate.

What leads for the future come out of these consideration? These are purely speculative, are not meant to be taken seriously as suggestions for manipulating childhood behaviour, but are of scientific interest. If dopaminergic stimulation improves MBD, then would *L*-dopa coupled with a peripheral decarboxylase work, or bromocryptine? Would *L*-tryptophan plus a MAO inhibitor be active since in animals these drugs produce 'serotonergic' stereotypy? Can the ventral tegmental syndrome be used as a model on which to screen drugs for the treatment of the MBD syndrome? Are the hyperactivities in rats produced by isolation or lead ingestion similar in any way to the ventral tegmental syndrome and by extrapolation, to the MBD syndrome, and if so is dysfunction of the A10 pathway of meso-cortical dopaminergic neurones involved? If indeed dysfunction of the A10 dopaminergic neurones is disturbed in the MBD syndrome, what is the cause? Conceivably, this could be a maturation defect, a genetic defect, due to perinatal insult, or just a 'normal deviant' in function. It seems to me that even if one considers the MBD syndrome in many otherwise normal children merely a behavioural problem falling within the bounds of normality, from the point of view of the neurobiology of behaviour, the actions of amphetamine and the data culled from relevant animal experimentation do suggest that children who behave in the way defined by MBD syndrome, behave in this way because their brains are different from other children's and that this difference might be explained by a primary or secondary difference in the way certain dopaminergic neuronal tracts function.

Summary

The hyperactivity syndromes produced by pharmacological means in animals are considered in the light of the actions of amphetamine and methylphenidate. The action of amphetamine which is considered most important in its effect in the minimal brain dysfunction syndrome is that of producing stereotyped behaviour. The behavioural syndrome in rats produced by lesions in the ventral tegmental mesencephalon consists of increased activity and disorganised behaviour and certain features of this syndrome respond to amphetamine administration, in particular the increased activity lessens. Again, this could be explained on the basis of amphetamine stereotyping behaviour. Perhaps, therefore, in minimal brain dysfunction one of the main features is the inability to attend to the task in hand. If this were the case the action of amphetamine in producing stereotypy would be to enable the child to concentrate on specific tasks. This idea is expanded by consideration of other animal hyperactivity syndromes.

Acknowledgement

I am very grateful to Drs. *Sahakian* and *Robbins* for allowing me to see their paper on the behavioural actions of amphetamine before publication. I am also very grateful to Dr. *Glowinski* for drawing my attention to the work of Dr. *Le Moal,* and to Dr. *Tassin* for allowing me to see the papers of *Le Moal et al.* (1977) and *Tassin et al.* (1977) before publication.

References

Grahame-Smith, D.G.: Studies *in vivo* on the relationship between brain tryptophan, brain 5-HT synthesis and hyperactivity in rats treated with a monoamine oxidase inhibitor and *L*-tryptophan. J. Neurochem. *18:* 1053–1066 (1971).

Green, A.R. and Grahame-Smith, D.G.: The role of brain dopamine in the hyperactivity syndrome produced by increased 5-hydroxytryptamine synthesis in rats. Neuropharmacology *13:* 949–959 (1974).

Green, A.R. and Grahame-Smith, D.G.: Effects of drugs on the processes regulating the functional activity of brain 5-hydroxytryptamine. Nature, Lond. *260:* 487–491 (1976).

Heal, D.J.; Green, A.R.; Boullin, D.J., and Grahame-Smith, D.G.: Single and repeated administration of neuroleptic drugs to rats. Effects on striatal dopamine-sensitive adenylate cyclase and locomotor activity produced by tranylcypromine and *L*-tryptophan or *L*-dopa. Psychopharmacology *49:* 287–300 (1976).

Hess, S.M. and Dopfner, W.: Behavioural effects and brain amine content in rats. Archs int. Pharmacodyn. Thér. *134:* 89–99 (1961).

Iversen, L.L.: Dopamine receptors in the brain. Science *188:* 1084–1089 (1975).

Jacobs, B.L. and Cohen, A.: Differential behavioural effects of lesions of the median or dorsal raphé nuclei in rats: Open field and pain elicited aggression. J. comp. Physiol. Psychol. (1975).

Jacobs, B.L.; Mosko, S.S., and Trulson, M.E.: The investigation of the role of serotonin in mammalian behaviour; in *Drucker and McGaugh* Neurobiology of sleep and memory (Academic Press, New York, in press, 1977).

Le Moal, M.; Stinus, L.; Simon, H.; Tassin, J.P.; Thierry, A.M.; Blanc, G.; Glowinski, J., and Cardo, B.: Behavioural effects of a lesion in the ventral mesencephalic tegmentum. Evidence for an involvement of A10 dopaminergic neurones; in *Costa and Gessa* Advances in biochemical psychopharmacology, vol. 16 (Raven Press, New York 1977).

Millichap, J.G.: The hyperactive child. Practitioner *217:* 61–65 (1976).

Randrup, A. and Munkrad, I.: Pharmacology and physiology of stereotyped behaviour. J. psychiat. Res. *11:* 1–10 (1974).

Rylander, G.: Stereotypy in man following amphetamine abuse; in *Baker* The correlation of adverse effects in man with observations in animals, p. 28 (Excerpta Medica International Congress Series No. 220, Amsterdam 1971).

Sahakian, B.J. and Robbins, T.W.: Are the effects of psychomotor stimulant drugs on hyperactive children really paradoxical? Med. Hypotheses (1977).

Sahakian, B.J.; Robbins, T.W., and Iversen, S.D.: α-Flupenthixol-induced hyperactivity by chronic dosing in rats. Eur. J. Pharmacol. *37:* 169–178 (1976).

Sahakian, B.J.; Robbins, T.W.; Morgan, M.I., and Iversen, S.D.: The effects of psychomotor stimulants on stereotypy and locomotor activity in socially-deprived and control rats. Brain Res. *84:* 195–205 (1975).

Sauerhoff, M. and Michaelson, I.A.: Hyperactivity and brain catecholamines in lead exposed developing rats. Science *182:* 1022–1024 (1973).

Sroufe, L.A. and Stewart, M.A.: Treating problem children with stimulant drugs. New Engl. J. Med. *289:* 407–413 (1973).

Tassin, J.P.; Stinus, L.; Simon, H.; Blanc, G.; Thierry, A.M.; Le Moal, M.; Cardo, B., and Glowinski, J.: Distribution of dopaminergic terminals in rat cerebral cortex. Role of dopaminergic mesocortical system in ventral tegmentum area syndrome; in *Costa and Gessa* Advances in biochemical psychopharmacology, vol. 16 (Raven Press, New York 1977).

Thornburg, J.E. and Moore, K.E.: The relative importance of dopaminergic and norabenogic neuronal systems for the stimulation of locomotor activity induced by amphetamine and other drugs. Neuropharmacology *12:* 853–866 (1973).

Valzelli, L.: The 'isolation' syndrome in mice. Psychopharmacologia *31:* 305–320 (1973).

Wender, P.H.: The minimal brain dysfunction syndrome. A. Rev. Med. *1975:* 45–62.

D.G. Grahame-Smith, MB, PhD, FRCP, Professor of Clinical Pharmacology, MRC Clinical Pharmacology Unit, University Department of Clinical Pharmacology, Radcliffe Infirmary, Woodstock Road, *Oxford OX2 6HE* (England)

Adv. biol. Psychiat., vol. 1, pp. 96–105 (Karger, Basel 1978)

Minimal Brain Dysfunction Syndrome and the Plasticity of the Nervous System

H.F.R. Prechtl

Department of Developmental Neurology, University Hospital, Groningen

Statement of the Problem

The role which structural damage and dysfunction of the nervous system play in the aetiology of childhood psychiatric symptoms in the so-called minimal brain dysfunction syndrome is still far from being clear with existing opinions surrounded by controversy. For obvious reasons neuropathological examinations of the brains of MBD children do not exist. Even if such specimens were available, it would be very hard to know what pathologists should be looking for. Therefore, all suggestions for brain involvement in the behavioural symptomatology are indirect and restricted only to signs of neural dysfunctions which may or may not be causally related.

There may be another source of evidence which could shed light on the present problem. In this paper a hypothesis will be put forward which connects findings of behavioural sequelae resulting from early brain lesions in animals with the behavioural symptomatology in MBD children.

The so-called MBD syndrome is characterized by enormous inter-individual variability. Furthermore, intra-individual symptoms vary greatly in different situations. They also show great changes during the course of development. The question arises whether this may be due to the phenomenon which has been called 'plasticity of the nervous system'. Although this term is ambiguous it covers also the fact that a damaged nervous system possesses a number of compensatory processes which may sometimes have an adaptive effect. During the last few years an impressive body of neurobehavioural studies has been produced concerning the difference between the sequelae of early versus late lesions. As a general rule it is apparent that the damaged nervous system has a larger capacity for compensation the younger the organism. There are, however, exceptions to this rule. Most of the work which will be reported here has not been designed as an animal model for the MBD syndrome but had other aims.

Great caution is therefore necessary in extrapolating from animal experiments to the human situation because of the well-known species differences in the mature nervous system itself and also in the kind and speed of maturational processes. There are, however, a number of phenomena which are found to be very similar in a large variety of species and they may therefore be also present in the human. The pre- and perinatal brain damage in the human fetus and infant is rarely circumscribed but is mainly diffuse in contrast to the localised surgical lesions made experimentally in the animal infant. The multiple lesions in the infant, however, may not have different mechanisms of compensation from the ones found in the animal experiments.

Unilateral Lesions and Their Compensation

One of the classic examples of compensation for early unilateral lesions is the work by *Kennard* (1936, 1938, 1940, 1942, 1944). She did not find any disturbances of motor development after unilateral lesion of the motor and pre-motor cortex if it was carried out in the first days of life. Bilateral lesions, however, could not be compensated. Interestingly enough the young unilaterally operated animals behaved normally 24 h after the operation and were not different from their control animals. Even their palmar-grasp reflex disappeared in the contralateral hand at the same time as on the ipsilateral side.

Similar results have been obtained from other species, especially the rat. In contrast to the severe handicaps found in adult rats after hemispherectomy, rats which have been hemispherectomized during their first days of life do not show any impairment later on. These early operated animals develop a strong ipsilateral cortical-spinal tract which compensates for the defect (*Hicks and d'Amato,* 1970; *Castro,* 1975). It seems, however, that the ipsilateral corticospinal tracts make somewhat different synapses on the ventral horn cells than would normally be the case (*Leong,* 1976). It is very important that a similar phenomenon, namely a hypertrophy of the uncrossed pyramidal fibres, has been also described in the human after early damage of one hemisphere (*Scales and Collins,* 1972).

A similar compensatory mechanism of the crossing system has been shown for the optic tract. *Lund and Lund* (1973) have investigated the degeneration patterns in the superior colliculus and lateral geniculate body after removal of one eye. If the enucleation was carried out in newborn rats younger than 10 days the remaining eye projected to the ipsilateral subcortical visual centre which was desafferentated by the original enucleation. This compensation was lacking in animals older than 10 days. This age dependency has also been described by *Guillery* (1972) in cats. *Lund and Miller* (1975) have studied the ipsilateral projection after eye damage in fetal rats. They also reported an innervation of subcortical visual centres by the ipsilateral intact eye.

Unilateral entorhinal lesions at 10 days in rats lead to an innervation of the denervated hippocampal dentate gyrus from the contralateral entorhinal area. There is neurophysiological evidence for the function of this abnormal innervation. However, it is possible that in this particular case the anomalous connections may be functionally maladaptive and they may disturb recovery.

Other examples of a takeover of denervated structures are fibre-sprouting from the intact side of the corticorubral projections (*Nah and Leong,* 1976) and also the aberrant bilateral projections from the dentate and interposed nuclei are given by *Lim and Leong* (1975), who said: 'The results showed that, aside from projecting to the contralateral red nucleus and nucleus ventralis lateralis, the efferent fibers of the dentate and interposed nuclei were seen to deflect at the decussation of the superior cerebellar peduncles and terminate in the ipsilateral red nucleus and nucleus ventralis lateralis.' The common denominator in all these studies is probably the defect in the normal interaction of crossing fibre systems at their decussation. It is obvious that a reinnervation from the intact side may lead to unusual and wrong wiring in the nervous system. On the other hand the outgrowth of a compensating corticospinal system may prevent a crippling condition, if the lesion was acquired early enough.

An exciting discovery was made by *Schneider* (1970, 1973), after neonatal unilateral lesion of the tectum in the Syrian hamster. The tectum is responsible for the orienting response to a lateral visual stimulus, e.g., food. If the superficial layers of the superior colliculus were destroyed on one side axons from the eye contralateral to the lesion reached the area of early damage, but also formed an abnormal decussation, crossing the tectal midline to terminate in the medial zone of the unimpaired colliculus. Hamsters with such an abnormal innervation showed wrong-direction turning in a response to visual stimuli in a large part of the visual field.

Lesions of Sensoricortical Areas

A series of studies has dealt with the problem whether functions may be spared after early lesions while lesions of the same areas lead to severe defects in the adult animal. Learning of auditory discrimination in cats depends on an intact auditory cortex. After bilateral destruction two different sounds or sounds of different duration can no longer be discriminated. However, if the lesions were made between the 7th and the 10th day after birth no deficits were found after training at the age of 6 months (*Scharlock et al.,* 1963). Similarly bilateral lesions of the somatosensory cortex in cats impair the ability to discriminate the roughness of the surface. If animals were operated neonatally, they were able to be conditioned to respond to such differences at the age of 6 months (*Benjamin and Thompson,* 1959).

Comparable results have been found for the visual cortex. Lesions of the visual cortex in the adult cat impair the placing response and visual pattern discrimination. If the ablation was carried out perinatally the lesioned animals were, after several months, no longer different from their controls (*Wetzel et al.*, 1965). *Murphy et al.* (1975) demonstrated that ablation of the visual cortex in newborn cats does not lead to a complete degeneration of the neurones in the lateral geniculate nucleus. These spared neurones may be involved in pattern discrimination in infant operated cats.

Early Lesions of Subcortical Structures

Bilateral destruction of the amygdalae and the periformic cortex, produces in adult cats and monkeys the dramatic effects of the so-called Klüver-Bucy syndrome. They consist of changes in emotionality, food intake, and sexual behaviour (*Klüver and Bucy,* 1939; *Kling,* 1966). If both amygdalae were destroyed in cats in the first weeks of life, several defects did not occur and others appeared only months later to a slight degree. *Kling and Green* (1967) have carried out similar experiments with the rhesus monkey. The neonatally operated animals did not show the reduction of anxiety and flight behaviour which is characteristic if the animals are operated upon as adults. Neonatally operated animals behaved normally 6–12 h after the lesion when they are given back to the mother in, for example, clinging and sucking. The further development of behaviour is unimpaired and neither apathy nor hyperkinesis has been observed. Later studies (*Thompson et al.*, 1969) have shown, however, that this is only true with certain restrictions if animals are tested in different situations. Early operated monkeys were later more nonchalant to normal stimuli if they were tested in their familiar cage. They were more anxious against their mates in the group and the social flight behaviour was not only maintained but rather increased. Such behaviour is perhaps due to a decrease in agression, which leads to a lower place in the social hierarchy.

An interesting group difference between normals and monkeys operated during the first 2 months of life was shown when they were tested at 3 years during a long stay in the test cage (*Thompson,* 1969). The amygdalectomized animals were significantly more hyperactive and cornering more than the controls. They switched more frequently between these behavioural patterns when they were brought into the test cage. If both groups stayed for 24 h in the same cage, these group differences disappeared. After 24 h, however, a new difference appeared. The operated animals explored more by chewing objects in the cage than the control animals did. These differences would never have been found in short-lasting experiments.

Another subcortical brain area is the septum which has been studied in respect to differences in the sequelae of juvenile and adult lesions. *Johnson* (1972) operated the septum in 7-day-old rats and compared their behavioural development with unoperated litter mates. The 'emotionality' of the operated animals was increased but remained constant during the first 90 days, while the control animals developed emotionality more gradually. Operated animals explored larger areas in an open field test compared to the unoperated controls. In the first 63 days they were hyperactive which then turned into hypoactivity as is known from adult animals after septum lesions. Of special interest was the result with learning experiments using an avoidance test in a two-way shuttle box.

All animals with septum lesions, irrespective of age in which the septum was destroyed, learned more quickly and efficiently to solve the task. They made more social contact in the open field situation than the control animals. Septum lesions, even if they are made in the 1st days of life, were not compensated. There were symptoms (hyperemotionality) which were only shown during the early age, probably before sexual maturity. Furthermore, conditioned responses may be carried out better after septum lesions. Brain lesions, therefore, do not necessarily deteriorate behaviour in all situations.

Another principle which can occur after early lesion in the nervous system has been studied by *Devor* (1975, 1976). The author made lesions in the lateral olfactory tract containing the efferent axons from the olfactory bulb which ends in the broad cortical field in the ventral forebrain. The intactness of the olfactory system in the male hamster is a prerequisite for mating behaviour. If the lateral olfactory tract axons were totally cut in hamster pups the proximal end of the axons branched widely in the neighbouring area, terminating on an area which they normally do not innervate. If, however, the tract was not completely cut but a number of fibers had been spared, then these intact fibers became branching collaterals and invaded the normal area of destination. The branching, however, was not sufficient to reinnervate the complete area of denervation and the farthest distal parts of the projections field lost their normal innervation. It seems, therefore, that there is a limitation to the total arborization per neuron, which can indeed compensate partly by innervating a vacated field but this capacity is limited by a form of conservation of total arborization available to each axon. In addition, this capacity is restricted to the early age of the animals, because it was not found in older hamsters.

An example of failure in a compensation of early lesions was provided by *Lawrence and Hopkins* (1972, 1976). In a rhesus monkey the corticomotoneuronal connections are gradually formed post-natally and reach the adult density at approximately 8 months of age in the rhesus monkey. Parallel with this development goes the maturation of discrete distal finger movements. If the pyramidal tracts were bilaterally lesioned at an age from 5 days to 4 weeks after birth, no 'relatively dependant finger movements' were developed during the surviving time of 3 years. Although these animals look clinically rather normal, the defect becomes obvious in specific tasks, for example in picking a peanut out of a small food well.

The Frontal Lobe

Since the study by *Akert et al.* (1960) the frontal lobe has been studied in rhesus monkeys with great intensity. I do not want to go into details of the many reports, some of them with conflicting results, because this area has recently been extensively reviewed by *Goldman* (1975, 1976). Only two points may be mentioned here, because they are of special interest in relation to our problem. The dorsolateral cortex seems to be involved in the behavioural problem of solving delayed responses. Ablations of this area in adult monkeys lead to a complete loss of the ability. If this cortical area, however, is lesioned in infant monkeys they do not show any impairment of the delayed response, at least not within the 1st years of life. Later on they may get into troubles at the age of 2 years. The conclusion was that at the early age subcortical structures are involved, and only later on does the cortex take over this task so that if it is lesioned the defect becomes manifest. Interestingly enough, there is an enormous sex difference in the effects of frontocortical lesions of the orbital prefrontal cortex. While delayed response performances were impaired at $2^1/_2$ months in males operated on as infants, females showed the same difficulties only at the age of 15–18 months (*Goldman et al.*, 1974). Recent morphological studies have not revealed any anatomical explanation (personal commun., by Prof. *Nauta*).

Beside this very interesting sex difference found in the effect of early lesions, the study by *Kling and Tucker* (1967) was revealing because if a lesion was made in the head of the caudate nucleus in addition to the frontal cortex, the delayed response was missing in 7- to 14-month-old animals. In addition, the postoperative behaviour of these animals was severely disturbed. Apathy, poor sucking, impaired grasping and temperature regulation, together with hypokinesis and epileptic fits, led to a rejection of these baby monkeys by their mothers. They had, therefore, to be handreared and showed later the behavioural defects of isolated reared rhesus monkeys described by Harlow.

Many other studies could be mentioned which have focussed on the effects of early lesions in the frontal lobe cortex on learning behaviour, using mainly the delayed response and Wisconsin General Test apparatus. Very little is known about the general behaviour of these animals. The omission, however, was rectified somewhat in a study by *Bowden et al.* (1971). The monkeys had been operated on the 47th to 52nd day of life and some received an orbital lesion, while others had ablated the dorsolateral cortex. At the age of 10 months the behaviour was studied with video recordings using 40 different behavioural categories; the animals were compared with non-operated controls. The animals with orbital lesions showed more differences in comparison with the controls than those with the dorsolateral lesions. The orbital animals were hypokinetic in the social situation. They showed half of the activity of the normals in contrast to the hyperkinesis in the single cage where they spent 72% of their time in locomotion (39% in the normals). Behaviour directed to the environment such as looking to the food well or grasping the wire was diminished in both operated groups. This study shows clearly how much behavioural characteristics of lesioned animals are bound to the specific context of study.

Mechanisms of Compensation during Development

The aforementioned examples are only a small selection out of the large material which has been published over the last decade or so on plasticity of the nervous system. For further details the reader is referred to a more complete discussion of this topic in publications of symposia including discussions such as: *Stein et al.* (1974), *Eidelberg and Stein* (1974), Experimental Neurology (1975), *Vital-Durand and Jeannerod* (1975), and the article by *Goldman* (1976). A number of conclusions can be drawn from these researches such as: distinct brain lesions in young organisms have different sequelae from lesions in adults. The nature of the mechanisms which lead to a greater capacity for compensation are not well understood. A few aspects, however, are evident. Cortical lesions may show different effects in the young animal compared to the adult because the cortex is simply not yet functioning and does not show defects after damage at least until the cortex reaches the maturational stage when it takes over functions from subcortical regions. Furthermore, fibre systems which are still growing may compensate more easily than fibre systems which are fully grown. Sprouting and branching are well-documented mechanisms which occur in the young infant animal but are not restricted to earlier ages and have been documented in lower adult mammals. Striking similarities to clinical findings have been shown by lesions of the caudate nucleus where the well-known syndrome of acute brain impairment observed in intensive care units for babies has been simulated in monkey. There is also the phenomenon of the latent periods, which is clinically manifest in human newborns in the form of acute neurological symptoms which disappear completely and may lead later to symptoms, in which other neurological defects are present. Also sex differences in relation to early lesions should be mentioned, which is daily experience in clinical observations in the human. Certain defects become manifest in particular situations but not in others: there is no general syndrome of brain damage but there are specific defects related to specific lesions which become manifest only in particular situations. There is also the striking effect of rather complete compensation of severe damages of brain structure by morphological restructuring of the growing brain. A restriction must be made, however, that not all compensations in the function are due to morphological rewiring as there is the possibility that damaged animals may solve the same problems via different strategies involving different brain mechanisms.

Although one can never be sure how much of these phenomena found in animal experiments are only analogous or homologous to the human situation, the striking similarities as described in this paper may indicate that similar mechanisms may be present in the human. One thing, however, we can be rather sure about, is that if a nervous system becomes structurally damaged at an early age it may grow via several morphological compensatory mechanisms into a different brain and this aspect may be one of the most important conclusions from these studies. Infants who acquire brain damage may develop a brain which is biologically different from the normally developing brain. The large variety of compensatory mechanisms, depending on the specific brain structures involved, may explain the large variety found in children with minor brain dysfunction. It also indicates that persisting neurological defects may not always be present but rather inconsistent behavioural deviations may be the only sequelae of large structural defects in the nervous system. The aberrant rewiring of the nervous system may not always lead to a brain with a specific defect, leaving the rest intact, but rather may produce a biologically different nervous system with peculiar properties in behaviour. Returning to the opening statement made in this paper it should be clearly borne in mind that deviant behaviour does not in itself signify a deviant brain structure.

References

Akert, K.; Orth, O.S.; Harlow, H.F., and Schiltz, K.A.: Learned behaviour of rhesus monkeys following neonatal bilateral prefrontal lobotomy. Science *132:* 1944–1945 (1960).

Benjamin, R.M. and Thompson, R.F.: Differential effects of cortical lesions in infant and adult cats on roughness discrimination. Expl Neurol. *1:* 305–321 (1959).

Bowden, D.M.; Goldman, P.S.; Rosvold, H.E., and Greenstreet, R.L.: Free behaviour of rhesus monkeys following lesions of the dorsolateral and orbital prefrontal cortex in infancy. Exp. Brain Res. *12:* 265–274 (1971).

Castro, A.J.: Ipsilateral corticospinal projections after large lesions of the cerebral hemisphere in neonatal rats. Expl Neurol. *46:* 1–8 (1975).

Devor, M.: Neuroplasticity in the sparing or deterioration of function after early olfactory tract lesions. Science *190:* 998–1000 (1975).

Devor, M.: Neuroplasticity in the rearrangement of olfactory tract fibers after neonatal transection in hamsters. J. comp. Neurol. *166:* 49–72 (1976).

Eidelberg, E. and Stein, D.C.: Functional recovery after lesions of the nervous system. Neurosc. Res. Progr. Bull. *12:* 191–302 (1974).

Experimental Neurology: Growth and regeneration in the central nervous system. *48/3:* part 2 (1975)

Goldman, P.S.: Age, sex and experience as related to the neural basis of cognitive development; in *Buchwald and Brazier* Brain mechanisms in mental retardation, pp. 379–392 (Academic Press, New York 1975).

Goldman, P.S.: Maturation of the mammalian nervous system and the ontogeny of behavior; in *Rosenblatt, Hinde, Shaw and Beer* Advances in the study of behavior, vol. 7, pp. 1–90 (Academic Press, New York 1976).

Goldman, P.S.; Crawford, H.T.; Stokes, L.P.; Galkin, T.W., and Rosvold, H.E.: Sex-dependent behavioral effects of cerebral cortical lesions in the developing rhesus monkey. Science *186:* 540–542 (1974).

Guillery, R.S.: Experiments to determinate whether retinogeniculate axons can form translaminar collateral sprouts in the dorsal lateral geniculate nucleus of the cat. J. comp. Neurol. *146:* 407–420 (1972).

Hicks, S.P. and D'Amato, C.J.: Motor-sensory and visual behavior after hemispherectomy in newborn and mature rats. Expl Neurol. *29:* 416–438 (1970).

Johnson, D.A.: Developmental aspects of recovery of function following septal lesions in the infant rat. J. comp. Physiol. Psychol. *78:* 331–348 (1972).

Kennard, M.A.: Age and other factors in motor recovery from precentral lesions in monkeys. Am. J. Physiol. *115:* 136–146 (1936).

Kennard, M.A.: Reorganization of motor function in the cerebral cortex of monkeys deprived of motor and premotor areas in infancy. J. Neurophysiol. *1:* 477–496 (1938).

Kennard, M.A.: Relation of age to motor impairment in man and subhuman primates. Archs Neurol. Psychiat. *44:* 377–397 (1940).

Kennard, M.A.: Cortical reorganization of motor function: studies on series of monkeys of various ages from infancy to maturity. Archs Neurol. Psychiat. *48:* 227–240 (1942).

Kennard, M.A.: Reactions of monkeys of various ages to partial and complete decortication. J. Neuropath. exp. Neurol. *11:* 289–310 (1944).

Kling, A.: Ontogenetic and phylogenetic studies on the amygdaloid nuclei. Psychosom. Med. *28:* 155–161 (1966).

Kling, A. and Green, P.C.: Effects of neonatal amygdalectomy in the maternally reared and maternally deprived macaque. Nature, Lond. *18:* 742–743 (1967).

Kling, A. and Tucker, T.J.: Effects of combined lesions of frontal granular cortex and caudate nucleus in the neonatal monkey. Brain Res. *6:* 428–439 (1967).

Klüver, H. and Bucy, P.C.: Preliminary analysis of functions of the temporal lobes in monkeys. Archs Neurol. Psychiat. *42:* 979–1000 (1939).

Lawrence, D.G. and Hopkins, D.A.: Developmental aspects of pyramidal motor control in the rhesus monkey. Brain Res. *40:* 117–118 (1972).

Lawrence, D.G. and Hopkins, D.A.: The development of motor control in the rhesus monkey. Evidence concerning the role of corticomotoneuronal connections. Brain *99:* 235–254 (1976).

Leong, S.K.: An experimental study of the corticofugal system following cerebral lesions in the albino rats. Expl Brain Res. *26:* 235–248 (1976).

Lim, K.H. and Leong, S.K.: Aberrant bilateral projections from the dentate and interposed nuclei in albino rats after neonatal lesions. Brain Res. *96:* 306–309 (1975).

Lund, R.D. and Lund, J.S.: Reorganization of the retinotectal pathway in rats after neonatal retinal lesions. Expl Neurol. *40:* 377–390 (1973).

Lund, R.D. and Miller, B.F.: Secondary effects of fetal eye damage in rats on intact central optic projections. Brain Res. *92:* 279–290 (1975).

Murphy, E.H.; Mize, R.R., and Schechter, P.B.: Visual discrimination following infant and adult ablation of cortical areas 17, 18 and 19 in the cat. Expl Neurol. *49:* 386–405 (1975).
Nah, S.H. and Leong, S.K.: Bilateral corticofugal projection on the red nucleus after neonatal lesions in the albino rat. Brain Res. *107:* 433–436 (1976).
Scales, D.A. and Collins, G.H.: Cerebral degeneration with hypertrophy of the contralateral pyramid. Archs Neurol. *26:* 186–190 (1972).
Scharlock, D.P.; Tucker, T.J., and Strominger, N.L.: Auditory discrimination by the cat after neonatal ablation of temporal cortex. Science *141:* 1197–1198 (1963).
Schneider, G.E.: Mechanisms of functional recovery following lesions of visual cortex or superior colliculus in neonate and adult hamsters. Brain Behav. Evol. *3:* 295–323 (1970).
Schneider, G.E.: Early lesions of superior colliculus. Factors affecting the formation of abnormal retinal projections. Brain Behav. Evol. *8:* 73–109 (1973).
Stein, D.G.; Rosen, J.J., and Butters, N.: Plasticity and recovery of function in the central nervous system (Academic Press, New York 1974).
Thompson, C.I.: Time in test cage and behavior after amygdalectomy in infant rhesus monkeys. Physiol. Behav. *4:* 1027–1030 (1969).
Thompson, C.I.; Schwartzbaum, J.S., and Harlow, H.F.: Development of social fear after amygdalectomy in infant rhesus monkeys. Physiol. Behav. *4:* 249–254 (1969).
Vital-Durand, F. and Jeannerod, M.: Eye movement related activity in the visual cortex of dark-reared kittens. Electroenceph. clin. Neurophysiol. *38:* 295–302 (1975).
Wetzel, A.B.; Thompson, V.E.; Horel, J.A., and Meyer, P.M.: Some consequences of perinatal leions of the visual cortex in the cat. Psychon. Sci. *3:* 381–382 (1965).

Prof. Dr. *H.F.R. Prechtl*, Instituut voor Ontwikkelingsneurologie, Academisch Ziekenhuis, Oostersingel 59, *Groningen* (The Netherlands)

Adv. biol. Psychiat., vol. 1, p. 106 (Karger, Basel 1978)

Closing Remarks

I will try not to abuse the last moments left to draw some conclusions from the various contributions. It seems quite clear that the MBD syndrome is not to be considered as a diagnostic entity or as a single disease, but rather encompasses a variety of subgroups of children with or without brain disabilities. *Kalverboer* has retraced for us the history of the concept of MBD, which has been influenced by psychogenetic theories as well as neuropsychological thinking. He has also discussed for us, as has *Yule,* the methodological problems involved in defining, assessing and evaluating the MBD syndrome. We have heard from Dr. *Yule* a comprehensive and critical discussion of the various psychological assessment procedures for diagnostic and treatment purposes and he has made some constructive proposals for refining these procedures.

The role of neurological assessment has also been underlined by *Touwen,* who has shown the importance of the developmental approach in discriminating between MBD and minor neurological dysfunction. A relationship between some neurological impairment and the behavioral syndrome seems to be present, but its significance is not yet clear in light of the obvious environmental influence on the child's behavior.

Prechtl has shed some light on the subject from the neuropathological and neurophysiological point of view and he has shown us that postlesional compensation is an important adaptive mechanism in the animal and probably the human brain. Concerning animal studies, *Grahame-Smith* has elegantly discussed the relevance of animal models to the understanding of MBD in terms of neuropharmacology and drug treatment, and has emphasized the importance of dopaminergic neurones. However, inference from animal to men is always a venture and there is apparently no ideal drug for the treatment of MBD, the most commonly known drugs being the central nervous stimulants, as has been described by Dr. *Pick.* Drug treatment is not the only therapeutic approach however, since we should not forget that what we label MBD is also a learning disability, which requires educational and psychological support, some investigators even proning behavioristic attitudes. Finally, *Shaffer* has made a significant contribution to the subject by underlining the need for controlled follow-up studies to learn more about the natural history of the MBD syndrome and by emphasizing the role played by social, familial and other environmental factors, a concept close to the threshold model of stresses interacting with some genetic predispositions.

In conclusion, we are dealing with a typical problem requiring a multidisciplinary approach and there is obviously a need for greater knowledge and more convincing studies.

J. Mendlewicz, MD, PhD, Chairman

Subject Index